MAR   2013

Heartbreak YOGA

Heartbreak Y♡GA

Learning to Survive and Thrive
Through Yoga, Meditation, and Laughter

AMY V. DEWHURST
Foreword by Sara Ivanhoe

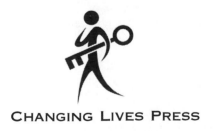

CHANGING LIVES PRESS

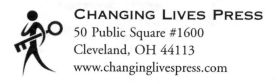

CHANGING LIVES PRESS
50 Public Square #1600
Cleveland, OH 44113
www.changinglivespress.com

Library of Congress Cataloging-in-Publication Data is available through the Library of Congress.

Editor: Shari Johnson
Cover and Interior design: Gary A. Rosenberg

Heartbreak Yoga logo designed by Zoë Kors
Heart Organ (page 6), heart dividing symbol (page 11), Chakra Girl (page 15), and Hanuman (page 246) by Larissa Hise Henoch
Heart chakra image (page 13) by Paul Heussenstamm
Yoga photography and cover photo by Kelli McCarty
Dancing Nataraj (page 86) by David Young-Wolff
Author photo by Rafaela Hess
Cover and yoga model: Jo Newman

Printed in the United States of America

10   9   8   7   6   5   4   3   2   1

Contents

Part III YOGA

With deepest love,
gratitude, laughter and tears,
in celebration, sadness and memory
of my beloved friend,
Chris Miller.

I love you more than
words can tell.

xo

Foreword

**Sara Elizabeth Ivanhoe, Master Yogi, Scholar,
Celebrity Wellness Coach, TV Personality**

Venice Beach, California • May, 2008

"Sooooo, why do you think you'd want to work for a yoga instructor?"

"Well, I've been working in the film industry for years and I just want something more meaningful, something . . . I can't really explain it."

"Uh, huh . . . ?"

"I know I don't really have experience in your field, but I'm a fast learner."

"Ok, well, do you like dogs?"

"Love them. Oh, she's so cute! What's her name?"

"Agatha. Aggie. You can call her Ag."

"Ag. Hi, Ag. I'm Amy. Awww—Ag. Schmag. Can I call her Schmag?"

"Do we have a choice?"

In the yoga world, we call it a "Lila." The Sanskrit word "Lila" essentially means "play." The word can refer to watching a play, being playful, or my favorite—when the gods are PLAYING with you.

A few hours earlier, a 27-year-old, hot, blonde Venice surfer chic went into her production job a little too tired and hung over and just snapped. She was, as we say "over it." When the boss headed out to a meeting, she scanned the internet for job postings and came upon one for a yoga instructor needing help running her business.

"How hard could that be?" she asked herself. "A yoga instructor? You mean get paid to sit around stretching? Sign me up! That job is mine."

"But it says here that you must love dogs—you're allergic," the friend at the next desk jealously rained on the parade.

"I'll fake it. I'll keep that smelly thing away from me, it'll be gone within months. You watch. I'm giving my notice tomorrow."

The "Lila" joke was on her. If she had known what she was getting herself into, she might never have taken the first step. Who would have known that not only did she become magically un-allergic to dogs, but that Agatha would become her best friend, co-worker, and the catalyst for her heart cracking open. Somehow once it felt safe to love a dog . . . the flood gates opened. (Turns out that Ag is not really a dog, but a Bodhisattva in a dog's body—we tricked Amy.) If she had known that she would become an embodied yogini and dedicated to the practice and study of both the physical and philosophical aspects of yoga, she might have said "Um, no thanks. I think I'll wait for a promotion to production manager and my own parking spot." Whether it was the gods playing a trick, or just "her path," down the rabbit hole Amy went.

We are so lucky that she did.

Everyone has their own "How I came to yoga" story. And although yours might not be quite as circuitous as Amy's was, you took the first step for a reason. If you've picked up this book, you're probably experiencing some sort of pain or grief right now. The bad news is that there is no magic pill to make it all go away. (Okay, there actually are several of them, but if you're reading this, it means you're looking for another way.) Yoga is not a cure, but it has helped millions of people for thousands of years navigate all forms of disappointment, rejection and heartbreak.

Whether your wound is old or fresh, whether you have been doing yoga for years or have never said the words "downward facing dog"— this book is for you. It is a vulnerable recount of one woman's journey that will have you laughing, crying and hopeful that you too, can pick yourself up, dust yourself off—and learn to love again.

Heartbreak Yoga includes a balanced yoga routine with beautiful pictures and detailed instructions on how to practice safely. It gives tips on eating healthy, holistic medicine, meditation and breathing techniques. Amy has called on the yoga community to chime in on the topic of love and has assembled a delicious mixture of inspiring quotes, songs and images—surely ONE of them will get through to you. As we say, "all it takes is one" for it to matter.

Worldly successes rarely feel as good as they are supposed to, but watching Amy grow into a compassionate, loving young woman, has been one of the most rewarding parts of my life. I still find it hard to comprehend that the Tween that flipped her hair in my living room, interrupted my sentences, said "Yeah I got it," and was "JUST FINE" all the time wrote a book called *Heartbreak Yoga*. It is a Lila—this time the gods are playing a trick on ME.

After a long writer's retreat away, Amy just came back to Los Angeles to finish up the book and start a new production job. She teaches yoga to the people in the office, brings healthy food to them for lunch, and is free to creatively chime in with her "yoga wisdom" on creative projects and day-to-day operations.

As the Zen saying goes:

"Before enlightenment—chop wood, carry water.

After enlightenment—chop wood, carry water."

For the home stretch of writing this book, we once again curled up on the couch where I made her wear socks and drink hot drinks. We called on Ag to help us edit, format and make Ujjayi Breath jokes. It's good to be back. I can now safely say with a smile . . .

My work here is done.

Sara Elizabeth Ivanhoe
Santa Monica, CA
January 2013

Pranams to Those Who Made This Moment Possible

Sri Sri Mata Amritananadamayi Devi
Danny Ducovny
John & Claire Dewhurst
Laura Amazzone
Vanessa-Ma Harris
Mukti Silberfein
Sridhar Silberfein

The Heartbreak Yoga Team
Photographer: Kelli McCarty
Models: Jo Newman & Paul Teodo
Yoga Tech Advisor: Brianna Welke
Ground Support: Zoë Kors, Craig Garfinkle, Eimear Noone,
    Heather Reinhardt & Mariel Hemingway

For the Love & the Lessons
Shari Johnson, Francesca Minerva, Ellen Ratner, Barbara Kopple, David
Cassidy, Larissa Henoch, Carol & Gary Rosenberg, Robert P. Williams,
Jon Dadbin, Chris Montgomery, Dan Horton, Jim Phillips, Karyn
Dilworth, Nanci Done, Lee Runchey, Kevin DeSoto, Alison Mason,
Kare Morelli, Robert Schnitzer, Craig Kessler, Richard Hernandez, Joe
Boiadjian & Marla, Samantha Whidby, Cody, Bella & Flower Silber-
fein, Noah P. Christensen, Durga Das (David), Mira, Tulsi & Han

Newman, Brett Mazurek (DJ 3rdi), Neem Das (Chris Morro), Radha Baum, Shiva Baum, Dana Min Goodman, Dan Steinberg, Govindas, Radha & Malachi Rosen, Zach Leary, Cosibella Cristenas, Kripa Robb, Karen Felice, Ana Maria Arumi, LA & NYC Amma Satsangs, Bhagavandas, Ram Dass, Krishna Das, Paravati Marcus, Denise Kaufman, Chani-Ma Nicholas, Mary Arden Collins, Mark & Bodhi Gorman, Nina Rao, Arjun Bruggeman, Genevieve Walker, David Nichtern, Devadas, Jeremy Frindel, Mark Whitwell, Kia Miller & Tommy Rosen, MC Yogi, Nick, Amanda & Mo Giacomini, Doug E. Fresh, Jai Uttal, Wah! Sarah Thompson, Terri Seiden, Kim Surowicz, Jennifer Quail, Jessica Lustgarten, Chris "Boyband" DeAngelis, Tudor Jones, Matt McNeill, Tim Frylinck, Jon Tortarella, Matt Mason, Chris "Coney Island" Vendetti, Local Zeros, Amanda & Eric Borja, Annie & Sean Gessell, Janet & Jerry Zucker, Alan Loeb, Donny, Lydia Silverman, Jamie Wright-Holding, Denis O'Sulivan, Jesse Toledano, Dan Cone & 363 Films, Matt Gordon, Lisa Barrett, Jenny & Norman Ollestad, Selena Palmieri Gable, Sharon Funke, Dawn Bridgewater, The Carey Family, The Baker Family, The Anthony/ Thomas/Jones Family, Justin Cohen, Les Koll, Shakuntala & Lolli, Bud, Michele Esrick, Meghan Kennedy Townsend, Gary Deutschman, Brody McHugh, My Lunch Table, Gina Podley, Carrie Grossman, Mandy Ingber, Perrey & Murray, Pete DeYoung, Evan Ross, Tracy Colombus, Tom Schey, Patti Hawn & Steve Middledorf, Suzanne Inez & Lalania Hudson, Gigi Gaston, Margot Dougherty, Catherine Soliman, Diane Antonia, Shima Razavi, Kadi Rodriguez, David & Julie Zucker, Richard B. Lewis & The Lewis Family, Gaby Jerou & The Tabak Family, Kirsten Sheridan & The Sheridan-McDonald Family, Susan, Jim Jim, Emma & Ava Murphy, Gerald & Francine Torino, The LaForge/Lucey Family, The Murphy/Owens/Madigan Family, The Heinzinger/Myers Family, Kim Seidler and The Seidler Family, The Kulesz/Lanni Family, The Terilizzis, The Fitzpatrick Family, The Landis Family, Annie Frylinck & The Frylinck Family, Kerri Tortarella & The Tortarella Famliy, Nicole & Mike Sandberg, The Sandberg Family, Cyndi Smith Taltry, Doug Corbett, Chris Byrne, Owens, Bernard, Johnny, Sabella, Wondra, Eidschun, Ilg, and The River Dell Starting

Line Up, Cynthia & Ara Khoriozian, The Carberry Family, The Rodriguez Family, Travis Eliot, Zach, Jorie, Liam, Kaia & Quinn Gallagher, Peter, Birgitta, Jake & Danny Breen, Kerri Branin, Melissa Halverson, Jean Pesce, Diana Jackson & Jamie O'Keefe, The Kuehne Family, The Quail Family, Nick, Vernoy, Jessica & Nicole Paolini, Dana Pustetta, Jay Burke, Mike Ponce, DJ Goldberg, Lisa Burgess, Annie Dickson, Beautiful Sarah Ivy, Miles Catalano, Dr. David Haberman, Deepak & Lana Ramapriyan, Brick Wallace, Evan Weinstein, Lee A. Hutton, III, Sylvia Allen, Karthik Dhandapani, Thomas Joseph Tobin, The Miller Family, The Weiner- Family, Aggie-Ji Ivanhoe, Vernoy Joret, Swanini Krishnamrita Prana, The 90291, The Bhakti Fest Family, The YogaWorks Family, Bhakti Yoga Shala, The First Congregational Church of River Edge, Sri Neem Karoli Baba, All the saints, guides and gurus on the path before, during and after, and of course . . .

Sara Elizabeth Ivanhoe.

(All roads lead home.)
Jai Ma!
Xo

*"I wish I could show you when you are lonely or in darkness,
the astonishing light of your own being."*

—HAFIZ, 14TH CENTURY PERSIAN MYSTIC POET

Introduction

HEARTBREAK IS THE WORST.

If someone told you that sticking needles in your eyes would alleviate the pangs of misery bellowing in your low belly, it would be pincushion city faster than you can say, "heal." Humans are the only species to engage in mating rituals for any reason other than procreation. The Museum of Natural History Department of Systematic Biology estimates there are between three and thirty million species living on the planet. We are among the ELEVEN who attempt monogamy. Our fellow mate-for-lifers include swans, lobsters, wolves, French angelfish, turtledoves, gibbons, black vultures, albatrosses, prairie voles, bald eagles, and termites.

I wonder how many termites sit at home on Friday night chomping on take-out pinewood, crying to Celine Dion's "My Heart Will Go On."

"But the Save-the-Dates already went out!"

"Pass the support beam appetizer, will ya?"

The anguish of heartbreak has brought us *Casablanca,* Led Zeppelin riffs and seasons one through ten of *Friends.*

We give guys our numbers, e-mail addresses and Facebook names. We text, flirt, pick out a new outfit, get ready for dinner only to be disappointed. We're bummed and home by the 11:30 p.m. showing of *Friends.* We tune in hoping Ross and Rachel will pull it together and just admit they love each other this time. But they don't.

So why do we do it to ourselves?

Why do we get back on the horse?

Why do we believe there are plenty of fish in the sea?

A lid for every pot?

And all the other underhanded cheerleads our loved ones pressure us with while RSVP-ing to black tie events?

"Is she bringing anyone special?" Don't you think if there were someone special I would have been invited "AND GUEST" ?!?

Let's admit it, Wonder Women of the new millennium, we do it because we know if we really want it, the right person is out there. We believe true love makes all the pain worth it and because at some point, every story has a happy ending.

It only takes one.

(Om.)

I am a Jersey Girl living in LA by way of New York City. This makes me the requisite recipient of the "I'm heartbroken can I come visit?" phone call. The terms and techniques contained within are the ones that have helped my TV-watching, beer-drinking, cigarette- smoking, chicken parm hero-eating girls and guys from back East. From within my Venice Beach apartment we have handled romantic heartbreaks, pink slips, and the emotional withdrawals of quitting white powdery substances, prescription pharmaceuticals and cigarettes. We even deep breathed through a "the wedding is off" text message (yes, a text message). I'm honored to have opened up my pullout couch and served digestible portions of organic granola and Guru Gita wisdom during their *commercial break*.

This book is a collection of stories, conversations, heartbreaks, lovemakes, the *ticker* and the hope that keeps us all going. There are approximately as many Ancient Allegories as there are pop culture references per page.

Like anything passed down over 5,000 years, there are infinite interpretations of these proverbs, lessons and yoga asana postures. The forthcoming are merely one woman's modern-day application of this wisdom, as she understands it.

Many of the terms you'll read are translated from Ancient Vedic Sanskrit. Hopefully you will enjoy the language lessons as much as I have.

Here's the first one: The word "Namasté" means: "The higher self in me, bows down to the higher self in you." There are many "riffs" off this greeting, including my favorite: "The light within me, sees the light within you."

Have you ever been to a Christmas Eve church service when *Silent Night* is sung in darkness? A single candle is lit off the altar flame. That single candle lights the candle of the person next to them, until that flame has traveled all the way around the sanctuary. Everyone "Oohs" and "Aahs," marveling at the renewed beauty this perspective provides.

Sometimes it takes a little darkness to see how much light surrounds you. Sometimes you need to be humble enough to hold out your candle, to see how many people support you. You would not have picked up this book if you weren't already glowing on the inside—if your candle was not meant to be lit.

You will get through this.

You are not alone.

You are stronger than you think.

The light within me, sees the light within you.

Namasté!

Amy

Xo

"Whatever comes to meet us,
know the darkness won't defeat us.
Stay strong, keep your faith alive."
—DAVID NEWMAN & FRIENDS

PART I

Heart

"Love is the strongest medicine.
It is more powerful than electricity."
—SRI NEEM KAROLI BABA (MAHARAJ-JI)

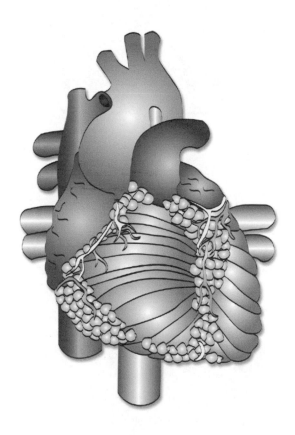

CHAPTER 1

The Physical Heart

"AME?"

"Yeah?"

"It's Dad. Mom had a heart attack. They don't think she is going to make it. She has four blocked arteries. She's in surgery now. The doctors are not hopeful. They said, . . ."

"What?!?! I'm getting on a plane. Will she be . . . ? She has to be! Dad, she has to be!"

"Ame, calm down. I don't know. All we can do now is pray."

My precocious "Law of Attraction"-loving self, suddenly wasn't so sure that our subconscious mind created every condition. I focused clearly on receiving good news upon landing. I pictured my mom well, making Thanksgiving dinner, decorating the Christmas tree, and my sharing with her every detail of every adventure, from whatever crazy corner of the universe I was calling collect from this time.

As I boarded the flight, I let go of my attempts to be in mental control of my mom's destiny. I prayed in earnest that whatever was best for her soul was what would occur. And that whatever occurred, I would be strong enough to survive.

One thing was for sure—I had to look in an old address book for God's phone number. It had been quite a long time since I reached out to that guy. Five years to be precise. One September he stopped returning my calls, so I stopped calling. I figured, *What's the point?*

He/She/It must have been surprised to be receiving frantic phone calls on every one of His/Her/It's lines. I was like an actor late for an audition. I called my *agent,* the *regular office* line, the *assistant's number,* the *studio's number.* I tried the *800 number* and when I didn't get through on any of those I tried God's direct dial, the bat phone used only for emergencies.

Hey, God, it's Amy Dewhurst. We met at the First Congregational Church in River Edge, New Jersey. I'm the one who narrates the Christmas Pageant every year. Oh, thanks. Yeah, it's fun. Everyone really enjoys it. We appreciate your blessing. Sorry I haven't been in touch lately. It's just I left you a bunch of messages in September of 2001, and I'm not sure if your assistant didn't pass them along, or maybe you called back and my voicemail was full or something? I never heard back from you, so I thought maybe I had done something to offend you, or you just weren't interested in me anymore.

Anyway . . . sorry to only call when I need something, but I was wondering if you could do me a solid? My mom, Claire, is in surgery. I'm pretty sure you two know each other. She was a deacon at the church, was in the PTA, worked full-time, made Sunday dinner for my entire family, making sure all the widowers left with a doggie bag. Yes, exactly! That's her. She is in surgery now. I don't mean to meddle, I'm sure you have a plan, but I've never really been great at minding my own business, so, if there's anything you can do, I would really appreciate it. And God, I'm sorry I let our relationship fade away. I'm sure your inbox was overflowing that September. Let's not let it go so long next time, huh?

This cycle of faith, doubt, mental focus and desperate prayers spun for six solid hours, from wheels up to wheels down, along the airport corridor and into my dad's poker face. I searched his eyes for answers. Never one to express emotion, he just nodded his head "yes."

Hey God, It's Amy Dewhurst again. We met at the First Congregational Church in River Edge. I'm the one who narrates . . . oh, okay, cool. I just wanted to say thanks for returning my call. I'm glad we're back in touch. Speak soon.

Six years later, I spoke with Dr. Richard Peterson about those six hours. While my hands were clasped in prayer at my heart, my mom's heart was in his hands, literally. Dr. Peterson is the thoracic surgeon who, in a code red, cut my mom's heart open, got out all the gunk, and sewed her back up—even better than new. The cartoon version of Dr. Peterson leaps around The Dewhurst Household like a lightning bolt, wearing medical scrubs and a red satin cape. The real man I met deflects these adulations, telling me "A quarterback is only as good as their team." In that analogy, Dr. P is the heart organ's Tom Brady, the obvious interviewee for the forthcoming inquiry:

Amy: What is the heart?

Dr. Peterson: The heart's job is really simple. It's a pump. It circulates blood throughout the body. The blood vessels pump blood through the lungs, to get oxygen, and it has to provide enough blood pressure in conjunction with the arteries to profuse blood to all your organs, your liver, your brain and all that. Then there's an electrical system that keeps the "lub dub, lub dub" [he imitates the sound of a beating heart] going.

Amy: Can you tell me what a thoracic surgeon is? What exactly you do?

Dr. Peterson: By the time I see people, they are all pretty much in dire straits. All preventive measures are gone. People mainly have blocked heart arteries, bad heart valves, cancer, or bad infection in the lungs. To overcome problems we repair heart valves or bypass heart arteries, or do both of those. You know from your mom, it's not a small thing; these surgeries are extremely invasive on the body.

Amy: Can you walk me through the process?

Dr. Peterson: Usually we cut into the chest, patient is asleep, obviously, we put the patient on a heart and lung machine and stop the heart, and then do whatever we are going to do—put in a valve or do a bypass, then start the heart back up again.

Amy: So let me get this straight, you literally rip the heart open?

Dr. Peterson: Yes.

Amy: Are Sita and Ram really in there? (Excitedly and unconsciously making a reference to *The Ramayana,* an ancient Hindu Epic, I spend a lot of time thinking about.)

Dr. Peterson: What's that?

Amy: Never mind. Can you tell me what is in the heart?

Dr. Peterson: Love of course! And blood vessels.

FUNCTIONS OF THE HEART AS AN ORGAN

- The role of the heart is to pump oxygen-rich blood to every living cell in the body.

- The human heart beats approximately 80,000 to 100,000 times a day and pumps almost 2,000 gallons of blood.

- In a person's life lasting 70 to 90 years, the heart beats approximately 2 to 3 billion times and pumps 50 to 65 million gallons of blood.

- It is made up of a muscle different from skeletal muscle that allows it to constantly beat.

- In order for the heart to deliver oxygenated blood to all cells, blood is pumped through arteries.

- Veins bring deoxygenated blood cells to the lungs, which then are oxygenated, and then sent back to heart.

- A continuous cycle keeps the heart pumping oxygenated blood and deoxygenated blood out to their designated destinations

    This is what is known as the circulatory system.

The Heartbeat

The heartbeat is made up of systole and diastole, which are the two stages of a heartbeat.

Systole: Stage when the ventricles of heart are contracting, resulting in blood being pumped out to the lungs and the rest of the body.

- Thick, muscular walls of both ventricles contract.
- Pressure rises in both ventricles, causing the bicuspid and tricuspid valves to close.
- Blood is forced up the aorta and the pulmonary artery.
- The atria relax during this time. The left atrium receives blood from the pulmonary vein, and the right atrium from the vena cava.

Diastole: Stage when the ventricles of the heart are relaxed and not contracting. During this stage, the atria are filled with blood and pump blood into the ventricles.

- Thick, muscular walls of both ventricles relax.
- Pressure in both ventricles falls low enough for bicuspid valves to open.
- The atria contract and blood is forced into the ventricles, expanding them.
- The blood pressure in the aorta is decreased, therefore the semi-lunar valves close.

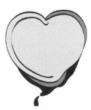

CHAPTER 2

The Heart Chakra

*"There is a light that shines beyond all things on earth,
beyond the highest, the very highest heavens.
This is the light that shines within our heart."*

—CHANDOGYA UPANISHAD

IN THE WISDOM TRADITIONS OF THE EAST—Hinduism, Buddhism and their denominations, the physical human body, the ten fingers, ten toes and everything they're connected to is called the gross body. Beyond that is the subtle body, the energy in and around the body. We might call it someone's "Aura," "Vibe" or even "Mojo."

The subtle body is reflective of the seven main energy centers of the body called "chakras." Directly translated, chakra means "wheel." It also means "turning" or "spinning." So these chakras, these energy centers in the body, are literally turning and spinning and having a grand ol' time; or, sometimes, they are sitting in the corner with their party hats on and crying because the boy they like asked a different girl to dance.

In this system, the "Heart Chakra" resides in the "Heart Organ"—the one I recently watched Dr. Peterson cut open from behind the observation glass. (And for all you *Ramayana* Fans, I'm pretty sure I *did* see Sita and Ram in there).

My friend Govindas built and cares for a temple, ashram and yoga school dedicated to the Heart Chakra. It is called Bhakti Yoga Shala. The programming serves the heart-based yoga heritage of Bhakti Yoga. Here, students learn yoga asana (physical yoga), meditation (mental attunement), kirtan (singing bhajans and mantra), satsang (community) and seva (selfless service). The Bhakti tradition dates back 5,000 years to India and made its way west to The United States on that cosmic wave called *Be Here Now,* the 1960s subculture classic book that *turned on* an entire generation.

In present day Malibu, CA, Govindas *tunes in:*

"The Heart Chakra is called the Anahata Chakra, which means the unstruck sound. Which is just this vast, eternal, unending space, and deep inside the heart chakra is what is called the hridayam. The hridayam is what the yogis recognize as the spiritual heart. Now it is in the heart chakra too that "atman," "the soul" lives in the heart. So, the heart is the center and in Bhakti yoga, we recognize the absolute center of the universe is the heart. Bhakti is called the path of heart. So we live through our heart. We play through our heart. We practice yoga from our heart. We live our lives from our heart."

The continued contents of that conversation contained his inquiry into my love life, an exchange of ideas about God, Guru, Self, bhakti elders, next generation seekers and concluded with taking a peak at his napping two-year-old son. If a sleeping baby's sigh isn't proof there is a God, I'm not sure anything is.

This contemplation inspired me to *drop out.*

I left my job as vice president of production at Mariel Hemingway's Film Company. I jumped on my yoga mat and wrote this book. I have never cared for relying on other people, so didn't want to wait for Dr. Peterson to leap in during a code red to get the gunk out of my heart. I knew I was strong enough and brave enough to do it myself. *You are too.*

"Go with your heart.
Your heart always knows . . . "
—GOVINDAS

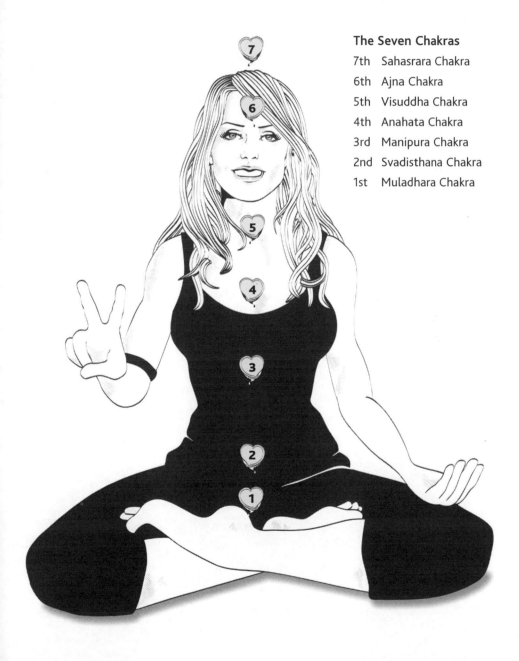

The Seven Chakras

7th   Sahasrara Chakra

6th   Ajna Chakra

5th   Visuddha Chakra

4th   Anahata Chakra

3rd   Manipura Chakra

2nd   Svadisthana Chakra

1st   Muladhara Chakra

PART II

Break

CHAPTER 3

That One September

"Brokedown Palace"

—THE GRATEFUL DEAD

IT WAS A TYPICAL, MIDDLE CLASS, SUBURBAN COMMUNITY smelling of freshly cut lawns. Behind picket fences were well-meaning but nosey neighbors and Detroit-built SUVs. The teens made out on church retreats, smoked spliffs on their way to varsity practice and sang Syd Barrett Songs as they aced the SATs. Proud parents snapped photos at prom parties, comparing curfews, report cards and whose virginity was still believed to be intact. Fourth of July Fireworks fell down on Memorial Fields as "The Boss" blasted from beer trucks. We were proud to be "Born in the USA."

There were the typical triple "our town" tragedies: horrific earth-shattering car accidents, awful overdoses and the stand alone suicide. This community came together in joy and grief like a Grecian epic, getting good at repurposing embroidered black funeral wear for Little Suzie's wedding just by adding a colorful wrap.

Then there was that one September when we perfected the skill. Our small pond police chief would go to Ground Zero to get the bodies, as Claire at Beaugard's would make a place for them to rest. The main street was short and the words were few. "Todd. Thursday." No one needed to say much more than that—time and funeral parlor location were well understood. I was working on Wall Street and going to school in the city. Based on proximity, willing creativity and the irrepressible urge to grieve optimistically, I took over "Celebrating the Life of . . ." collage duty. The college kids would comment on my compositions, coming home on weekends for wakes.

My group of Jersey Girls became like a team of professional, fashionable mourners, trading in our standard issue 20-something Steve Madden Shoes for more reasonable flats. The grief/heat combo of standing room only funeral services always concluded with a fainting or two. I observed early on it was the girls in three-inch-plus heels who had to lock out their knees to stand up straight that were usually the first to hit the floor. But who could blame them? They wanted to say goodbye to their first loves in style. "It's what he would've wanted me to wear," she said, uncharacteristically strong. We stood together sobbing as Scooter, her 20-year-old atheist, anti-establishment boyfriend's corpse was being carried out of the Catholic Church, draped in an American Flag.

First the leaves fell, then the snows came. Stockings were hung from the chimney with care, in hopes that "The Missing" would soon be there. New Years' Resolutions consisted of "Please God, if you bring _____ home, I promise, I will never _____ again." It was around Valentine's Day the DPW finally cleared the crowded commuter parking lot. If there was no DNA discovered, they would donate unclaimed cars to the fire department for "scared straight" DUI drills during driver's ed.

We buried empty caskets, and with them, mom and dad's dream that little John-o's job in the big city would afford him a slightly better life than they had had; an extra AC in the den, power windows & vacations "down the shore," even during leaner years.

Meanwhile, Back at Work . . . combat soldiers with uzis had been deployed downtown. The Bull and The Bear were barren. Subways, sidewalks, StairMasters and bar stools were all eerily empty. Government issued IDs allowed entry to the cobblestone streets of Old New York. There you would frantically search the faces of survivors striding past.

Desperate families would plead with handmade flyers, "Have you seen my dad/mom/husband/wife/brother/sister/son/daughter/lover/neighbor/

rabbi/priest/dog/cat/fiancé/ friend . . .?" A regretful shake of the head was the default response. You couldn't make eye contact with the families. You could barely breathe from the ever-escaping fumes.

There was a woman at The New York Sports Club who would ALWAYS take *my* treadmill during *my* assigned time. She would pretend she couldn't see me waving the sign-up sheet in her direction over her *Financial Times* newspaper. She would pretend she couldn't hear me shouting "Excuse me, your time is up!" over her Sony Discman tracks and StarTAC cell phone calls. She would pretend she couldn't respond, having just taken a big sip of Pepsi from the can. She would pretend she couldn't feel me tapping her shoulder. Of course not, she was winging her bony Rolex & Harry Winston-clad arms around trying to fling me off. I hated that bitch and her gorgeous red Kate Spade bag. She loathed me, Miss PYT, probably 30 years her junior, flagging around the stupid treadmill sign-up sheet, indignant about time.

Her tycoon husband had left her for a younger woman before I had even been born. She learned to day trade out of divorcée defiance, victoriously taking over 51 percent of his brokerage firm. You know what they say about a woman scorned—she joins the boys' club at Harry's in Hanover Square and smokes Cuban cigars just a few minutes after burning the bras. She felt, despite NYSC standards, she was entitled to the extra fifteen minutes of cardio at my workout's expense. "Show some respect for your elders!" she spewed.

That ornery old bitch was one of the first recognizable faces I frantically scanned in early October. With overwhelming relief, I fell into her ugly old chicken-arms. I cried grateful but silent sobs, as she wailed aloud, "Thank God you are okay, I have been looking for you everywhere, I knew you commuted on the PATH Train, I thought . . . Oh God, Sweetie, thank God you are ok. Thank you God. Thank you God. Thank you God."

But that story was just one in a million (1 in 2,997, to be more precise). Never again did I see the funny, sweet guys from Fire Company #5 who teased me each time I emerged from the World Trade Center's basement mall, Banana Republic bag in hand:

"Uh, Oh, somebody didn't make it home laaaast night."
"Woo-hoo, walk of shame shopping trip."
"Hey Bertolino, your girlfriend's cheatin' on ya."
"Ah ha ha ha . . ."

The homeless woman who slept on the steps of Trinity Church:
"Alms for the poor? Thank you. God bless you."

Gloria, the woman who worked at Mangia Deli, who took the lunchtime delivery orders over the phone:
"Amy, Kerri & Dan? One twenty Wall Street, right? The usual for you guys?"

My personal trainer Blythe:
"One more rep, you can do it, I believe in you . . ."

My friend Todd:
"Hey, I'm going to make the 7:14 train, can I grab ya a Heineken for the ride home?"

My friend Jen's dad, Mr. Fialco:
"Give your old man a call. Tell him I'll drop ya home on my way. Save 'im a trip to the train station."

And many, many, many more . . .

What wasn't conveyed in those overused images of the towers tumbling down was the innate silence the city suddenly fell under. Well, that and the smell. I'm not brave enough even to begin a description of the smell. A re-watch of "Schindler's List," "Born on the Fourth of July," or "Glory" may help you imagine it. Sucking in dry wall dust during a renovation might help you breathe it. Add to that the paranoid fear of a cop driving behind you after you've had three glasses of wine at dinner, or the way your hair stands on end in historically spooky spaces—Alcatraz, Amityville, Auschwitz. There. That's the zygote of a description. I'm braver than I thought. *You probably are too.*

I tell you this grim tale not as a victim, but as a survivor of earth-quak-ing, building-breaking, heart-shattering, soul-squeezing, mind-numbing, God-questioning, wholly humbling, totally vulnerable, on-my-knees, "How could this have happened?" heartbreak. Some forthcoming melo-dramas may have seemed hysterical and ungrounded otherwise.

With love and respect to all who survived, and especially to those who didn't, I'm grateful to have had the following experiences. I missed my train that Tuesday morning.

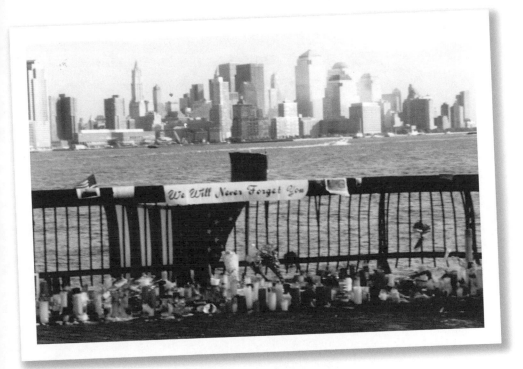

"My City of Ruins"
—BRUCE SPRINGSTEEN

" . . . When I think back to that time, I was so sure someone must have the answer. I wanted someone to tell me how to make my life-pain free. Looking back, I can't imagine who I thought got through their entire lives and managed to avoid the pain. Now I realize there is not now nor has there ever been a single person on this planet who has successfully avoided the pain of being a human.

"Pain is part of the deal."

—GURMUKH KAUR KHALSA

CHAPTER 4

Grief

PHASES OF GRIEF

1. Denial
2. Anger
3. Bargaining

4. Depression
5. Acceptance

EFFECTS OF GRIEF

Effects of Grief on the Physical Body

- Exhaustion
- Fatigue
- Muscle tightness or weakness
- Aches and Pains
- Restlessness
- Can't sit still
- Insomnia
- Unable, or not wanting to get out of bed

- Sleeping too much
- Disturbing dreams
- Loss of appetite
- Overeating
- Nausea
- Indigestion
- Intestinal disorders; diarrhea, excessive weight gain or loss
- Anxiety

- Headaches
- Shortness of breath
- Chest pain or pressure
- Tightness in throat

- Heaviness in throat
- Paranoia you could pass in the way in which your loved one did (disease, accident)

Effects of Grief on the Mind and Heart

Unpredictability of Emotions:

- You are laughing one moment, and crying, or unable to move the next.

Numbness:

- An initial period of shock and disbelief (this could be one week or usually up to a year). It allows the body to absorb the loss as is comfortable. After this denial wears off grief usually onsets in a full wave or sharp pain.

Sadness & Yearning:

- Overwhelming sadness and longing. Missing the physical closeness of your loved one.

Relief & Guilt:

- If the death of a loved one comes at the end of a long illness, or it was a conflicted relationship, there can be a sense of relief, quickly followed by guilt.

Regrets:

- "I should have . . ."
- "If only I had . . ."
- "He/She would . . ."

Anxiety, Worry & Fear:

- A helpless, panic-stricken feeling.

Mental Confusion:

- Trouble concentrating or completing tasks. A general forgetfulness, or inability to make decisions.

Anger:

- You may be mad at yourself, the loved one who has departed, the situation, disease, doctors, God, the world . . .

Effects of Grief on the Heart and Soul

- Anger at God
- Why did this happen?
- What was the purpose for this?
- Was this part of God's plan?
- What did I do to deserve this?
- What did he/she do to deserve this?
- What was the reason for this senseless death or loss?

Social Effects of Grief

- Withdraw socially
- Voluntarily isolate yourself
- Detachment
- Disinterest
- Lack of connection to previously loved activities, interest and even people

- Suspicion
- Irritability
- Hostility

OR

- Only engaging in social activities
- Fear of being alone
- Fear of going home
- Additionally: People whom you once felt close to or supported by are suddenly unavailable to you. They are unable to relate.

> *"The Lord is near to the brokenhearted*
> *and saves the crushed in spirit."*
> —PSALMS 34:18

CHAPTER 5

A Tale of Two Heartbreaks
East Coast—West Coast

IN THIS FIRST PERSON ACCOUNT OF BI-COASTAL HEARTBREAK, I swear to tell the truth, the whole truth and nothing but the truth. However, some names have been changed to protect the guilty. If you are enraged, please contact me privately circa cabbage night for egging addresses. No drive-bys.

BIGGIE

"As for lovers, well, they'll come and go too. And babe, I hate to say it, most of them—actually pretty much all of them are going to break your heart, but you can't give up because if you give up, you'll never find your soul mate. You'll never find that half who makes you whole and that goes for everything. Just because you fail once, doesn't mean you're gonna fail at everything. Keep trying, hold on, and always, always, always believe in yourself, because if you don't, then who will, sweetie? So keep your head high, keep your chin up, and most importantly, keep smiling, because life's a beautiful thing and there's so much to smile about."

— MARILYN MONROE

The notorious CJB or "Biggie," as we will henceforth refer to him was a hot popular senior at a neighboring high school. I was a freshman running around barefoot Sharpie-ing Grateful Dead Lyrics onto Converse One Stars while he dated adult women and drove fast cars. He was Mr. "2 Cool" from *Adventures in Babysitting* with bedroom eyes—even at 17. We met at a hotel party. Remember those? Someone's older brother rented a $69/night room at the HoJo and snuck in a 30-pack of MGDs? Boys left hung-over. Girls left hickied. Everyone reeked of stale cigarette smoke and Drakkar Noir. Chickenheads in booty pants came in and out of that room like a Beastie Boys Music Video audition line, laughing at lame jokes, trying to hold Biggie's glance a moment too long. They batted their eyelashes, bra straps and Blunt wrappers like they had heard the sweet sounds of Krishna's Flute. It was as entertaining as it was nauseating.

This medium-pretty girl in a tight orange T-shirt tried hard to win Biggie (and us) over. No one really took the bait, but no one turned down her offers to go get ice, open beers, or pack bowls either. In a drunk-on-one-wine-cooler teenage foreplay standard move, she started to kiss Biggie's neck.

All physical indications *literally pointed* to the conclusion that he was enjoying himself. So then why did he keep looking over at me?

Didn't he know I wasn't pretty?

Didn't he know all the boys at my school always liked all the other girls?

Obviously he hadn't had a clear gaze at my thighs yet; I better say something self-deprecating before he gets the wrong idea, thinks I am "good enough" and is actually interested.

Surely he couldn't still be looking at me.

But he was.

The next day, my friend Ali talked to her boyfriend, Bryan, who was Biggie's best friend. Bryan told Ali and then Ali told me that Biggie told Bryan that he thought I was cute. I squealed and told Ali that I thought Biggie was cute too! So, Ali told Bryan that I told her that I thought Biggie was cute too. So, Bryan told Biggie that Ali told him that I told Ali that I thought he was cute too. Biggie told Bryan to tell Ali to tell me that we should all hang out soon. Bryan told Ali that Biggie told him to tell her to tell me that we should all hang out soon. So, Ali told me that Bryan told her that Biggie told him that we should all hang out soon. Aaahhh!!!

And so the tension began—April 20, 1995.

Eleven years, 3,000 miles, and a million missed moments later, I was working as director's assistant on a studio feature film. The crew moved from New York City to Los Angeles "temporarily." I had been offered a promotion—a development executive position at a production company. I accepted. Signed a lease. Booked a flight east to empty my storage unit in NYC and make a real go of it in the Golden State.

My two-week itinerary was as follows:

FRIDAY:	Fly from LA to NY/NJ
SATURDAY:	Pack/ship storage unit
SUNDAY:	Fly back to LA
MONDAY–THURSDAY:	Wrap up last week of old job in LA
FRIDAY:	Fly To NY/NJ for best friend's engagement party
SATURDAY:	Best friend's engagement party
SUNDAY:	Fly back to LA
MONDAY:	New job begins in LA

I've never been great at planning ahead or remembering to use my frequent flyer miles. Ah well. Nobody's perfect.

Flight #1: LA to NY/NJ

I picked up my rental car and called my best friend, Sue.

"Screw it! I'm going to call him. I'm starting my new life; I don't always want to wonder 'what if?'"

"Good! Do It!" she replied, hoping this whole "California Thing" would blow over sooner rather than later, so we could commence with *her* plan of marrying, procreating and having our kids marry each other so we could officially become related (as though being best friends since you were three doesn't count as family). Peshaaaa.

Sue was newly engaged to a wonderful guy we affectionately referred to as "Jim Jim Murphy" due to his over-polite penchant for introducing himself as such. "Hi, I'm Jim. Jim Murphy." He had a nice firm handshake and class for days. Our dads love him.

I dialed Biggie. All the years of near misses came flooding back á la *An Affair to Remember* (or *Sleepless in Seattle,* for you youngsters).

He picked up on the first ring.

My heart leapt into my throat.

I talked fast.

He talked faster.

There was the notion of implied hand-gestures on either end of the phone.

We're Italians, we talk-a like this-a.

The conversation segued through a number of topics, never addressing that I was in town, wanted to see him (give up my career, marry him and have a hundred of his babies). The rental ride plowed down the main drag of Small Town USA to get to the bridge and into The Big Apple. As it did, I caught out of the corner of my eye, some hot guy, strolling in circles on his cell phone, waving his hands around in exaggerated gestures.

"I think I see you!"

"What!? Where are you?!"

"I'm on Kinderkamack, is that you?!"

"What are you doing on Kinderkamack?! I thought you were in California. Yes, that's me. Omigod. You're here."

I jumped out of the moving vehicle, *as* I threw it into park, "Yeah, I'm here."

He looked into my eyes taking it in. Saying slowly, "Wow. You're really here."

I looked back into his dark brown eyes, so deep I could have jumped in and stayed forever. "I'm really here."

"Finally," he said, grabbing me in a hooded Giants' sweatshirt-hug.

"Finally," I exhaled into his big, strong, safe, hot-guy arms. It's as though I had always belonged there. It felt brand new and like going back home all at once.

Ahhh.

I'm finally here and I will never leave again. Forget Paris. What more could I ever want than this embrace?

"Christaaaaphaaaaa."

My heart sank. *Nooooo.* I held my breath waiting to see what kind of hoochie momma was wrapped around the corner of the storefront. As we got older, the eyelash and bra-strap batters got more threatening. Four years his junior, Biggie and I spent a decade engaged in a comedy of Columbus Day errors, only seeing each other a few times a year in public places. Be it a wedding, funeral, Memorial Day barbeque or a random Thursday night we were both in town and at the local bar, Biggie was NEVER without some leggy broad on his arm. They were former models, special ed teachers who specialized in S&M, "tasteful" strippers from Scores, and that one girl who once dated Derek Jeter. (Ali and I snickered, "And by 'dated' surely she meant . . .")

The pattern went a little something like this:

We would see each other.

Our eyes would light up.

We would run toward each other like a soap opera montage, get all excited talking fast with our hands about nothing at all, touching each other every chance we got—and then when the pacing slowed and we stared deep into each other's eyes, about to admit something life altering, some girl who made it to the final qualifying round at the Playboy Mansion but was only hired as an alternate would put her perfectly manicured hand around his waist, signifying ownership. At which point he and I would ease into a conversation about the weather or whatever, trying not to lock eyes in a Tesla-powered storm.

"Chrrriiiissssttaaappphhhhhaaaaa."

No, please no. God no. Not again.

"Chrissstaaappphhhaaaaaaa."

Maybe if I don't look at it, it won't see me. Maybe it will go away. Go-go-gadget gamma-ray. Get 'er outta here.

"Chriisttttaaaapphhhaaaaaa."

"Whattt, Maaa?!"

"Ouuuuhh, sorry. I didn't know ya had company."

"Ma, you remember Amy . . . Dewhurst. The girl who . . ."

"Oooooohhhh yeeeaaaaah of course I remembah. Christapha talks about ya all the time. The movie stah out there in Hollyood, huh?"

Hardly.

Until this promotion I was a glorified coffee-fetcher, scraping by on minimum wage, crashing on my friend's couch in The Valley, while he "cooked" Raw Foods for the Red Hot Chili Peppers, but we weren't discussing details yet. I peeked up at Biggie. Never before has someone so tall, dark and handsome become so slouched, blushed and embarrassed. It was awesome. I immediately loved Biggie's mom.

The storefront my new best friend emerged from was "little Christapha's" side project, a boutique shop for vintage car parts. In other words, every guy's wet dream. As if his baller banker status and paid for in cash condo weren't enough, he had to have a cool hobby that made him money and friends too, right? Where else would you get a spark plug for a '65 Shelby and a cold Chimay in a chalice?

This kid had been balancing his checkbook since before any of us even knew how to balance our checkbooks. Or knew where our checkbooks were. Or if we even still had that account open. Or . . . well, it would just be easier to ask our dads for a twenty than figure out all that complicated banking stuff. "Daaaad, I'm going to the mall. Can I have . . . ?"

The next night we celebrated Halloween. Biggie was having a party (perfect!). We were all invited (perfect! perfect!) and there was enough room for us all to stay over if we couldn't drive home (perfect! perfect! perfect!).

Thriller blasted from brand new Bose speakers, paid for in cash, plugged into their own power strip far away from foot traffic. This medium-pretty girl in a tight orange cat costume tried hard to impress *James Bond.* He didn't really take the bait, but he didn't turn down her offers to go get ice, clean up the kitchen, or take out the trash either. In a drunk-on-ten-Jell-O shots, twenty-something standard foreplay move, the tight orange cat tried to kiss James Bond's neck, but James Bond had his eyes on another girl. He monster-mashed over to Malibu Barbie, locking the big browns on her.

I did fall in this time.

"Finally," he said searching my face, asking for an invitation.

"Finally," I said inviting him in.

He kissed me. "Ahhh, I've been waiting all week for that," he sighed.

"Me too." I nearly imploded with excitement.

"Really?"

I nodded my head yes. "Well, all week and ten years."

"Me too," he said looking like *he* might implode with excitement.

"Me three," said Sue looking like *she* might implode with excitement. Jim Jim Murphy pulled her away from our private moment.

And that's why Biggie loves him.

The rest of this evening and the following morning is censored for a PG-13 Rating.

Flight # 2: NY to LA

That week in LA, between flirty text messages and film screenings, I caught myself accidentally listening to the Lite FM station. The entire Michael Bolton catalogue suddenly became crystal clear. Have you heard of this Sade woman? She's really somethin'.

Flight #3: LA to NY/NJ

Biggie picked me up from the airport. All was amazing. Flowers, champagne, bubble baths, it was like a Mount Airy Lodge commercial come to life. From beneath the covers we planned the next 80 years "Till Death Do We Part," and all the other promises people make to each other without necessarily accepting the responsibility that comes with those words (or those intimacies).

Biggie pulled out his brand new Mac Book Laptop, paid for in cash and always kept in the case far away from liquids or table ledges. He booked his flight west for Thanksgiving. I booked my flight east for Christmas. We agreed that in the spring, one of us would move in with the other. He Googled real estate in LA. I Googled the pros and cons of The Northern and Southern Cross Country Car Routes.

"Well, if we go north we can hike the Grand Canyon. If we go south we can go to Graceland. "Let's flip a coin." I said excitedly.

"Let's check the weather reports and mileage it will put on the car," he said seriously.

I don't remember which way the coin landed because, he kissed me and then . . . this part of the story is censored for a PG-13 Rating.

The morning of Sue and Jim Jim Murphy's engagement party, we girls tied little white ribbons on anything within reach. Sue looked radiant as ever in her "I'm the bride" ensemble. There was something just breathtaking about this new version of Sue, something so stable and grounded. She had always been beautiful, but when Jim Jim Murphy walked in the room, she just lit up. And that is why *I* love him.

This evening had the potential to be one of the best nights of our lives.

What do you get when you add an Irish Catholic to an Italian Catholic? Forty-six IMMEDIATE family members, all of whom are named after the saints: Anthony, Nicholas, John, Peter, Paul, Jerome, Christopher, Mary, Theresa, Francine, Rosemary, Little Tony, Little Nicky, Johnny, Petie, Paulie, Jer, Little Chrissy, Mare, T, Frannie, Ro, The Nina, The Pinta, The Santa Maria . . .

If someone yelled "MA!" sixteen women turned their heads. If an ambulance drove past, forty-six people did the sign of the cross. To see Sue's dream coming true was absolute magic. I have never been happier.

Nor have I ever seen two merging families, better suited for one another.

The Maries, Frannies and Ro's couldn't wait to meet Biggie. The Little Nickys, Paulies, and Peties too.

"Ooouuuhh, what's he liiiike?"

"Should I grab 'im a drink? When is he comin'?"

"How do you know him?"

"When did you get togetha?"

"So what about this California job?"

"When is he comin'? The galamad is almost gone."

"I'll make 'im a plate, he should be here soon."

"Where does he live?"

"When are ya movin' back?"

"They give ya health insurance at that movie company?"

"He's comin' to the weddin' right? I mean, if you guys are goin' steady, maybe he'll even be in the weddin'."

"When is he comin'? The shells and gravy are almost gone."

"I'll make 'im a plate, I bet he just got lost. He'll be here soon."

I vacillated between thoughts of relief, *So, great—it's all settled then,* and the feeling I was being stuffed in a straitjacket, suffocated and forced to conform. The evening went on and soon the trays of ziti and kegs of Guinness were kicked. The bartender knew that empty glass = make another Cosmo. The girls knew to ask, "Is he here yet?" every time we made eye contact. The party was over and with it, the hope that Biggie would ride in on his white horse, or Black Nissan Pathfinder paid for in cash and hand washed every Saturday Morning with an infomercial-purchased shammy.

"Mare, you can throw out the plate you saved for Biggie."

The previously interested chorus of well-wishers now looked at me with pity.

"That's what she gets, thinkin' she can have it all," I heard one of them say. Like any of us would have chosen to juggle work, love, finances, physical fitness and two-income mortgages had we thought about it long enough. Where were the labor and delivery nurses, home ec teachers and Suze Orman, when that decision was made?

Flight #4: NY/NJ to LA

I woke up hung over, humiliated, heartbroken and dangerously late for my flight. I had a middle seat. Lucky me! I sat between an eager, green-eyed film studio internship applicant on the aisle and a talkative, animation house office manager-type at the window. Lucky me! Miss Window made herself sound important by using words like "Greenlit," "Lot" and "Commissary." Master Aisle naively kept asking her questions about greenlighting, the lot and the commissary. Lucky me! The inflight movie was *The Break Up*. Lucky me! I drowned out the misleading musings between the woman who ordered copy machine toner for a living and the poor kid who thought this was his big break, by watching *The Break Up*. Lucky me!

I became bummed for the kid who held on to that woman's business card like his life depended on it. He didn't know it now, but he was in the process of having his heart broken, too. By next week he would know this woman had wrapped blatant lies into her casual conversation using words like "studio brass," "the money people," "so and so over at la, la, la." He would have at least a million of these little heartbreaks once he stepped foot in Hollywood. One day he would look at himself in the mirror of his Porsche and that cute, ambitious smile would be gone. He'd snap at the valet, and catch himself carelessly using sentences like, "Well, her box office wasn't very good on her last movie. She means nothing." She means *nothing*?

I became bummed for the woman who was so unfulfilled she had to misrepresent herself. She obviously had grown a thick layer of protection over her lonely heart. If she had someone at home who paid any attention to her, or loved her just for who she was, she wouldn't have to pretend to know Robert De Niro just by calling him "Bob." Maybe if she had skipped the third mini-bottle of Beefeater on the plane, woke up fresh tomorrow and went for a run before ordering copy toner, she would have the confidence to sign up for one of those websites where people meet people, like Match.com, JDate or EHarmony. I'm sure she didn't want to have to rely on the attention of this poor little greenie to validate her existence. I'm sure she just woke up one day and it was 10 years, 20 pounds and 3, 650 boxes of 3-hole punched paper and 2-inch brads later. It happens.

I became bummed for Jennifer Aniston's character in *The Break Up*. Everyone has had the feeling: *This is it, you can exhale, everything will be okay now,* and then it's not. I became bummed for Jennifer Aniston. She has an Emmy, a Golden Globe, the stamina and skill to star in a sitcom for ten years, a great bod, great friends and a smile that lights up TV screens at 7, 11 and 11:30 p.m. nightly. Jennifer Aniston is a "10" and even *she* had her heart broken. Team Jen dignified the most public divorce since Princess Di and Prince Charles. When did all this get so complicated? What ever happened to "Happily Ever After"?

I crawled home to my brand new apartment overlooking the ocean. Just four days ago, this freshly-painted, 10 X 10 box was filled with love, light and the excitement of cooking Biggie a Thanksgiving Dinner. Now, it was cold, dark, small and sad. The fact that I only had a bed, a lamp and a surfboard suddenly didn't seem so cute and charming. It seemed immature and depressing.

Worse, my moving boxes hadn't arrived and the airport lost my luggage. Remember the promotion? *Just go to bed,* I thought. *It will all be magically better tomorrow.*

Before brushing my teeth and saying my prayers, I downloaded two pity party soundtrack faves: Bob Dylan's "I Can't Believe She Acts This Way" and David Allen Coe's "You Never Even Call Me by Name." It's amazing what you will cling to in a storm.

Monday morning my phone rang at 5 o'clock.

Yes! It's him. It has to be him.

Nope. It was my mom calling to congratulate me and wish me luck on the first day of my new job. She hadn't heard about the heartbreak *or* figured out the whole time difference thing yet, apparently.

I arrived at work early, set up my office, logged on to my new computer and looked for an email from Biggie. But there was no email.

The work phone rang. But it wasn't him.

I received a text message. But it was Sue.

The FedEx guy came to drop off a package. But it wasn't "I'm sorry" flowers.

Now, let's say you were dumped, are having a hallucination that there was probably a mix-up, and are desperate to hear from Mr. Right. Do you think that:

A. Your ten-hour workday would go fast or,
B. Your ten-hour workday would go by slower than the melting of molasses frozen with Walt Disney?

If you guessed B, you are correct. I wish I could offer you a prize, but as it turns out my paycheck, bonus, and moving stipend had actually NOT been directly deposited into my account yet. The two songs I purchased on iTunes had overdrawn my account and I would not be receiving that income until the next pay period, 15 days from now. And no, my petty cash reimbursement for $7 lattes for the director, producer, editor and homesteaded multi-millionaire musicians "_____" and "The _____" wouldn't come until then either.

I suddenly understood what Gloria Gaynor and squealing sorority girls since the 1970s had been carrying on about this whole time. When I started the "I'm sorry I told you to just get over your break-up I had no idea how bad it could be" phone calls to my girls back east, I spoke at length with Ali. Ali had recently walked in on her live-in boyfriend of five years having midday sex with their next-door neighbor. Afternoon de-nightmare.

Between bouts of depression and despair, I gasped for air. "I just can't breathe, it feels like there is a bag of bricks on my chest and shoulders."

In a quip more matter-of-fact than Janeane Garofalo reading the DOW, Ali replied, "Yup, that's what it feels like." As though this is common knowledge. Like EVERYONE had been through this. My eyes rolled. Nothing could be as bad as this. No one on the planet has felt this crushed; they don't understand.

As it turns out, a light poll of men and women I knew indicated that yes, in fact they did understand. The bricks-on-chest and/or punched-in-the-stomach feeling is standard and don't expect it to fade anytime soon either. My rogue romantic research also revealed that everyone from every socio-economic class, taste, style and geographic location has been through this. The average adult experiences three major heartbreaks throughout their lifetime. The question "Have you ever had your heart-broken?" was almost immediately followed by the words "Of course," then a loud groan—or, a loud groan followed by the words, "OF COURSE!"

You may think, "What's the big deal?" I'm not at all comparing this Biggie heartbreak to vacancy caused by the physical departure of a divorce, live-in lover or morbid loss. In my story however, Biggie is the "Big One." Serious boyfriends of whose hearts *I* have broken can cor-roborate this.

There are certain people you just have a spark with—who haunt the corners of your mind when you are tired or lonely. When you get the wedding invite and it DOES say "AND GUEST." The big "What If?" During the decade of near-misses, and even till this day, mutual friends will mention, "Biggie was just talking about you. He said he saw you in an episode of this, your name in the credits of that." I spent years casually slipping into the shore-to-shore catch-up calls: "Have you seen him? Was he with anyone?" There are just these people and it doesn't always make sense, and your brain knows better, but the fireworks have gone off, the birds are chirping, the bells are ringing and with all pomp and circumstance around you, it's nearly impossible to act rationally.

So I sat on my surfboard in the small but serene Ocean View apart-ment and made friends with my suffering. I didn't have any of the nor-mal life distractions. No friends, no family, no social obligations, no moving boxes, no money in my bank account, no nothing.

No return call.

No explanation.

No nothing.

"Wherever you go for the rest of your life, you're always in the middle of the universe and the circle is always around you. Everyone who walks up to you has entered that sacred space, and it's not an accident. Whatever comes into the space is there to teach you . . . Our life's work is to use what we have been given to wake up. If there were two people who were exactly the same—same body, same speech, same mind, same mother, same father, same house, same food, everything the same—one of them could use what he has to wake up and the other could use it to become more resentful, bitter, and sour. It doesn't matter what you're given, whether it's physical deformity or enormous wealth or poverty, beauty or ugliness, mental stability or mental instability, life in the middle of a peaceful silent desert. Whatever you're given can wake you up or put you to sleep. That's the challenge now: what are you going to do with what you have already—your body, speech your mind?"

—PEMA CHODRON, TIBETAN BUDDHIST NUN AND DIRECTOR
OF GAMPO ABBEY IN THE LINEAGE OF LAMA CHIME RINPOCHE
AND CHÖGYAM TRUNGPA RINPOCHE

THE HEARTBREAK YOGA INSTITUTE FOR RESEARCH AND INQUIRY LIGHT POLL OF MEN AND WOMEN I KNEW THAT INDICATED YES, THEY DID UNDERSTAND

Govindas—Bhakti Yoga Shala, Santa Monica, CA

Amy: Have you ever had your heart broken?

Govindas: Of course.

Amy: What was it like?

Govindas: Well, when our heart is broken we feel a separation from our divine beloved and there is separation anxiety. This is sort of the essence of what Bhakti is all about—this longing to be connected with our divine beloved. So when in our human relationships our heart is broken we feel that sense of separation and pain within our hearts. It's sort of a microcosmic reflection of that bigger sense of separation that we can potentially feel from the divine, from God, Guru, Self, The Universe, whatever you feel comfortable calling it; that "ONE" ness that exists within everything, within all of us, throughout all of creation.

Sharon Gannon—Co-Founder of Jivamukti, New York City, NY

Amy: Have you ever had your heartbroken?

Sharon: Yes many times and each time I felt separate and alone. When my heart broke I fell out of love—forgetting to remember the ever present-ness of love.

Amy: It's hard to remember when you can't eat, can't sleep, can't breathe. How do you even define something like love?

Sharon: God is love. Love is Oneness. It is from Love everything has come and back to love we are trying to go. Love is our true nature. Love is where all separateness dissolves. Love is all-inclusive. True love is unconditional and independent; it does not depend upon another, it is ever present—it is our ground of being.

Norman Ollestad—Novelist, *Crazy for the Storm*

"I stare at our bed. Three months prone, awake, without appetite, grappling her sudden departure. She left me in a day. I never saw it coming.

The initial shock should have passed by now, I rebuke, easing onto both knees. Falling on my face earlier tonight should have been rock bottom, the thud that ended my downward spiral. But I'm down on my knees, a terrible relapse."

Patti Hawn—Author, *Good Girls Don't*

"I shivered uncontrollably, and then something cracked deep inside my chest where he had just been. My sobs startled me; they were noisy and violent, and seemed to come directly from the void in my belly."

Anonymous Male Novelist

"I wasn't ready for it to end. I fought to keep us together. I fought for her. Until I realized one important thing: "Why would I fight for someone who didn't want to fight for me?"

Melissa Kirk—*Psychology Today* Blogger

"Heartbreak means facing the inevitability that everything we love will someday be gone from us."

Anonymous Amazing Woman Recently Dumped by a Douchebag I've Always Hated

Amy: I'm sorry, pup. Are you going to be okay? What can I do?

Anonymous amazing woman recently dumped by a douchebag I've always hated: No, I mean, I don't know, probably not. Maybe at some point. On the upside, I am going to be really skinny. I can't eat. I threw up everything I ate when I tried. I'm going to be well rested, because I slept for twelve hours last night and don't want to get out of bed. But I think I might have a cold, dark, heart now. I'm nervous I'm just going to be like dead on the inside forever.

Amy: You won't be dead on the inside forever—you won't live that long.

Anonymous amazing woman recently dumped by a douchebag I've always hated: (Laughs) Shuuuuut Uuuuuppp. You knooooow what I mean. I'm just nervous this feeling won't ever go away. What if I always feel this way?

Jesse Toledano—Filmmaker, 363 Productions

The things that make us who we are, that make us unique, we can think of like the gears of a machine. Heartbreak feels like those gears will be forever broken and that we will never work again. And it's not just that feeling of being out of sync but a feeling that the very components that define us are rotten at the core.

Love feels like those gears are working flawlessly, like they are set in a motion that has been perfectly designed, and that they will continue to work for all of time. Love has the power of taking those very components of us, the ones that are most vulnerable to darkness and doubt; love can make them feel like our greatest strength.

And unfortunately we cannot have one without the other. The depths of a broken heart are only felt if love shows us how special those parts of us are. We can never know how special they are until we know how much they can feel wrong.

Dr. David Haberman—Author of award-winning book, *Journey Through the Twelve Forests;* ACLS/SSRC NEH International Postdoctoral Fellowship; Fulbright-CIES Research Scholar Fellowship; Smithsonian-AIIS Senior Research Grant; Fulbright-Hays Fellowship for Research Abroad; Trustees Teaching Award (2002)

"We live in a time when we understand that the natural world is very threatened, VERY threatened because of us, right? And it could be that we are seeing, the unraveling of life as we know it on this planet, it could be. So that we could be living in a time when life is really dying on this planet. That opens up a whole different relationship with the world that we live in. It becomes very vulnerable. When lovers become vulnerable with each other there is a deepening of the love and I think that that is our moment. The beauty is still here in a way, but it's a threatened beauty, it's a vulnerable beauty. I think that is our relationship with things. Anyone who has lost a parent, who is attending a dying child, there's a special love there. There is such a beauty in that child, and yet you know that it could go one way or another. And to still stay open to that, that's the challenge, that's the real courage."

Jai Uttal—Grammy-nominated World Music Artist and Bhakta

"Love brings vulnerability and vulnerability can bring fear, so what do we do? Do we shut down the vulnerability and shut down the fear, so that we don't feel afraid? Well, certainly most of us, including myself, have done that. But obviously, our experiences show that that is not the best answer. So we move into the fear, and the humbling nature of that vulnerability and pray that we are protected and safe and that we can keep loving without running away from that helpless, scary feeling that love can sometimes bring to our hearts; and that way love grows, but it's not always a happy-go-lucky process—and yet, I wouldn't want any other process."

Jean Pesce—Lead Singer/Jean & The Geraldines, Williamsburg, Brooklyn

Getting my heart broken made me feel like The Velveteen Rabbit. I imagined my ex playing at the seaside with his new toy, while I was in a sack full of discarded shit waiting to be tossed into a bonfire. Except, when I shed a tear, no nursery magic fairy came to my side. And inside the sack weren't other discarded toys, but bourbon and cigarettes.

I decided to stay inside my dark, discarded sack, and just wait it out . . . until I could at least stop crying. I experienced unbridled despair and loneliness, the likes of which crippled me for unknown black stretches of time. I cried so hard for so long, that my eyes swelled shut permanently for about a week. Which isn't so bad. I know a girl who cried so hard, she broke a rib. I shit you not.

When I mustered the strength to crawl out of the sack, blinking at the daylight like some sort of pale, nocturnal cave dweller who had never seen the sun. I was determined to get laid and move on. But when one is still this swollen and raw, reeking of cigarettes, bourbon, and lament, you don't realize that you have changed forms.

When you're heartbroken, you wear it on your sleeve; it's all-consuming. You become hopelessly repellant and unpleasant, when you need someone the most. You involuntarily exacerbate your own grief and pain.

**Mary Firestone—Writer and founder of Wild Precious Life,
Los Angeles, CA**

"Of course! I was 16 and a new student at a new high school. At the
first school assembly, I clapped eyes on the student body president and
I was smitten. We dated for several months and I felt like I couldn't
believe how this amazing 'man' could adore me and want to be with me.
Well, after a school dance where I was introduced to Kahlua for the first
time and wound up in the infirmary busted, he didn't. He literally
dumped me in my little hospital gown with a wad of gum stuck in my
hair. What a spineless politician . . . and at such a young age! Not only
did I grapple with that hollow, gut wrench of heart break for several
weeks, I also had to endure a disciplinary meeting that he ran where he
doled out my punishment. It consisted of stuffing envelopes for the
Annual Fund and being at school for extended hours."

Jimm-i V.—Owner, the Venetian Surf Shop, Venice, CA

*"Shattered . . . in a frozen zone. I've stood alone as a stone,
in the middle of a river, time.
Observing it flow by, riding a perpetual low tide.
Pondering why.
Heart so torn, rip tides caused by, Richter scale shifts in my tectonic life.
Layers of strife.
A fault furrowed of mine for sure, my salt burrowed in time
to burn the bad memories in my mind.
Press the coal to diamonds.
For her, yes I."*

Masao Miyashiro—Old skool punk rock bassist, TONE DEF and Rated X

"I'm still here. Busted heart and all."

Anonymous Angeleno

"A broken heart will shine a light on all the things you hate about yourself and make them feel real."

Mariel Hemingway

Amy: What do you think heartbreak is?

Mariel: "Heartbreak is, well . . . oh come here, I love you, don't be sad. You're beautiful. His loss. (*We hug.*)

Mariel: It's happened to everyone.

Amy: Yeah right, I bet it's never happened to you."

Mariel: "Oh please, . . ." (*censored*)

Amy: But you're Mariel Hemingway! How could he do that to you?

Mariel: [She shrugs her shoulders.] I told you, it happens to everyone.

Bryn Chrisman—Yogamaya, New York City

"Of cooooouuurrrse I've had my heartbroken. On my birthday, December thirtieth, and then I had to teach a class at noon the next day. New Year's Eve. Aaaarggghhh!!!"

Kaycee Smith—Fishbone Music Management and Merch Girl Extraordinaire

"Heartache is somebody you thought you could trust with your life ripping your heart out. Leaving you alone, drowning in the worst pain you've ever known. Emptiness in your soul, ache so deep you never could have imagined anything hurting so bad."

Nicola Graydon Harris—Freelance journalist, broadcaster, writer, editor, *The Sunday Times Magazine, The Saturday Telegraph Magazine, The Daily Mail, Mail on Sunday, The Evening Standard, Eve, Marie Claire,* **and** *Harper's Bazaar*

Swan Song

I once heard my heart breaking. I was sitting by a loch in Scotland an hour before midnight on New Year's Eve. The water was perfectly still and a few feet in front of me a lone white swan floated luminous in the shallows. Tears were rolling down my face when suddenly there was this sharp cracking in my chest. It was so loud the swan turned its lovely head my way. My tears stopped as I thought, 'So that is what it sounds like when your heart is breaking.'

My boyfriend and I had planned a romantic festive season in a cottage on the banks of Loch Fyne. He was beautiful with dark hair and eyes like sapphires who knew how to cook miso soup. I thought he might save my life. Instead he broke my heart. But maybe that is one and the same thing.

My twenties were filled with controlling relationships but he was different. He gave me space, let me breathe and was present, listening and loving. There was a wildness in him too: when we were in nature, he inevitably leapt naked into lakes and waterfalls. More than once, we made love in open fields giggling as planes passed overhead. And when he made love, it was with an exquisite balance of tenderness and passion. This is it, I thought, this is The One.

But that Christmas Eve something snapped and the man I loved was nowhere to be seen. At a drinks party he turned violent over the choice of music and I dragged him out to the loch as small children shrank away. His sapphire eyes had turned black and he began talking in a cross between Elizabethan and gibberish. As our eyes got used to the darkness, two white swans emerged with their beaks touching and their long white necks forming the shape of a heart. 'Look,' I whispered, hoping their quiet grace would calm his frantic, strange behavior.

That week we spiraled into the darkness. More than once I found his hands around my throat. Sometimes he crawled into a ball and wept but mostly he spoke in riddles and his eyes just got blacker and blacker. I don't know why I didn't abandon him but I didn't. Then one day he took my car and disappeared. In driving rain, I paced the road, half mad myself, terrified he would turn up dead. That day I saw a lone black swan desperately paddling against the wind.

I called friends who called a friend who happened to be a doctor at a local mental health facility and a search party went out. He turned up in a pub, bare-foot, and gabbling. My car was found in a ditch several miles away. The doctor gently informed me that my boyfriend was manic psychotic and I had no choice but to have him sectioned. The drive to the hospital was the most painful I've ever had to take.

So there I was alone on New Year's Eve with the swan and my own breaking heart. The shock of it had stopped all emotion; instead there was this silence and something else; an expansion, as if something else had entered in.

Later, near dawn, a book at my bedside fell open at a quote by Rumi. It read, "Crack open my heart, Beloved, so that I might receive your Limitless Love."

Like I say, maybe, in breaking my heart, he had saved my life.

Jeremy Parker

Amy: What does it feel like?

(In the stylings of Sublime, LA's best beach band, Meet Me At The Pub's front man, Jeremy Parker just starts to serenade): "I tried to drink my blues away, they always come back the next day. I even tried a hundred girls. That was good for a one night thrill, but I miss you, yeah I do, I really miss you I'm so blue, 'cause I'm so lonely without you. I'm so lonely without you. My whole life's been about you. 'Cause I'm so lonely without you, wwwuuuu, ooouuuuhh, ooouuuhhhhh . . ."

Crash—Surfing Instructor

Amy: Have you ever had your heart broken?

Crash: Of course, Duuude. It suuuuuuuucks. Will you be my valentine?

Amy: No.

Crash: How 'bout now?

Amy: No.

Crash: How 'bout now?

Amy: Maybe.

Crash: Sweeeeet. Hop on my handlebars. I'll buy you a burrito.

And we rode down the beachfront bike path, off into the sunset . . . sorta.

Gil Fortis—Screenwriter

"When she left me, I was at a loss. I was paralyzed with indecision. I didn't know what to do or how to get over this feeling of abandonment.

"Then it occurred to me: I could finally get rid of all these stupid pillows."

RJN

(Screeching down Mulholland Drive under August's Blue Moon, my blue convertible served as a chariot for this world-renowned musician. An individual of VERY few decisively selected, soft-spoken words, but many masterful drum beats, I asked him the usual):

Amy: Have you ever had your heart broken?

RJN: Of course.

Amy: What was it like?

RJN: (*Loudly*) UGGGGGGGHHH!!

Amy: Whoa. That bad huh?

He silently nodded his head yes.

Amy: Can I quote you on that?

He silently nodded his head yes.

We never talked about it again.

Dr. Peterson—Thoracic Surgeon

Amy: "Do you think someone can die of heartbreak?"

Dr. Peterson: Yeah! I absolutely think they can and have. Their hearts are broken.

Amy: Have any of your patients ever died from heartbreak?

Dr. Peterson: Well, I often see older couples when they have been in relationships a long time, and one of them passes. Soon after, the other one, who had no preceding medical condition, they go too. What we call heartbreak, loss can certainly be injurious to your heart. It's not maybe; it's for sure. Everything is at the cellular level, but what bio-enzymatic process heartbreak directly affects, I don't think anyone can tell you exactly. Cells have memories. DNA memory at the basic level. Not necessarily in your brain, cognizant, but in the cells.

Amy: As I understand it, each cell of the body is like its own little computer, or its own little ecosystem.

Dr. Peterson: I think ecosystem is a better way to put it. It's not a brain, it's not like a computer, it's more an ecosystem that can be adaptive or destroyed. Look at viruses and how they affect cells. That's how cancer comes around—all the cells going crazy. But your body is set to defend itself. It's really incredible. Human beings are really incredible.

Amy: What are some of the ways the body defends itself against emotional stresses like a heartbreak?

Dr. Peterson: When people go through that they sleep more, their drive isn't there, they pull back. They're not as aggressive and there are changes that you make because your body just doesn't feel good. It protects itself. There are far more negative ones too, like stomach ulcers and diarrhea. Even having heart attacks. So, that's one.

Amy: My rogue observation of heartbroken "friends" is that the symptoms of heartbreak echo the symptoms of grief. Denial, anger, bargaining, depression, acceptance. Can't eat. Can't sleep. Can't breathe.

Dr. Peterson: Your "friends," huh? Well, that's interesting and very true. Right. Grief really puts a huge stress on your body. It just does. It's not good for you. It's not good for your GI Tract, your eating and digesting. It's not good for your blood pressure. You know, driving even— you're not as tuned in with your situation around you. It can be very dangerous.

Amy: Even deadly?

Dr. Peterson: [He laughs] Yes, Amy, even deadly. [Pause] So who was this guy?

Amy: Eh, not worth our time.

LOSS

"Yet, year after year, I find ways to hide. I've hidden from relationships under too many layers of fat. I've hidden from myself by getting wasted and watching TV instead of doing my creative work. I've hidden from my own needs by constantly caretaking others. Even knowing that the god/guru part of me knows my heart's desires, I foolishly try to hide. From what? Love?

"It takes an immense amount of courage to live in love, in truth, in openness. Even though I asked Maharaj-ji* for a pure heart and mind and for faith, I guess I forgot to ask for courage. Back then, I didn't know how much I would need it."

*Sri Neem Karoli Baba

—Parvati Marcus

I lost a very good friend of mine.

His name was Chris Miller.

Thirty-one years old. Married six months.

He was a caring, gentle sweet soul with the knowing eyes of Yoda.

A look from Chris could make all your worries melt away.

He was the kind of guy who would put his arm around you when you said you were "Good," but really you meant mad, sad, tired, upset, hurt, hungry—

Old grannies, babies, and dogs loved him.

So did I.

He was struck by a rare disease and died 72 hours later.

If my life were to cease at this exact second, I would be beyond honored to be remembered with the amount of laughter, tears and Mazzone's pizzas as Chris. He was an extraordinary being we are all so lucky to have known.

The hospital staff and Claire at Beaugard's remarked that they had never seen more people come to pay their respects in all their years. Even that one September. Now, 11 years older, this group of friends collectively has had children, bought houses, gone through divorces, buried parents and any other "Death and Taxes" reality life provided us with. But this just didn't add up. Nothing about this scenario was okay, or made sense. I couldn't find a silver lining anywhere in the collage-making process this time. The girls and I just cut and glued in silence. Complete shock befell us all.

This experience made us question our mortality. I cleaned up any loose end I ever had; mental, emotional, financial, spiritual. Sue and Jim Jim Murphy had wills drawn up to be sure their daughter, Emma, is always taken care of. Gross. When did we start talking like this? When did we become our parents? Somewhere in there it happened. We all grew up.

In doing so, we didn't numb out with beers at Beemer's Pub like we did that one September (and the subsequent winter months, until they finally cleared the commuter parking lot). We dealt with our grief like adults, talking and sharing in our experiences—thirtysomethings pondering the big questions.

This opened a floodgate for me.

I was healing. I hid out.

I watched every episode of Mad Men, went to the dentist, and called my niece ON her birthday (not a week earlier/later with some exaggerated "Sorry it's early/late" present in the mail). I went to the gym, 6 p.m. yoga classes, and watched the sunset. I live on the Pacific Ocean. Why don't I do this every day? That's why people move to the beach—duh. I cleared my schedule of superfluous coffees and "generals." In other words, I took a deep breath. I really went "In." I took care of ME.

If you haven't tried it, I sincerely recommend it.

TUPAC

The very first day I emerged from the cocoon, not yet knowing I was a butterfly, I met Tupac. We'll call him "TS" for short.

A city of transplants, there is a joke heard around agency assistant mix-ers and al-anon meetings alike: "No really, but where are you frommmm . . . ?" TS was actually frommmm here and had one of those glamorous/ tragic/interesting/public upbringings you read about in *People Maga-zine*. He was wonderful but guarded. Open but closed. Somewhere between has been, could be, and 'eh forget it.

I've never been attracted to someone so soft, smart or sad before. He reminded me of a beautiful pedigree bred from two Westminster Cup winners, but when they found out he had a limp, stopped feeding him the filet mignon and only changed his cage once a week. His parents' close friend, the artist formerly known as _____, played at their 50th Anniversary Party about 15 years ago.

After partying like it was 1999, TS and his cronies took the anniver-sary gift his parents had bought for themselves, a new Maserati, out for a "Smoke Ride." It was last seen wrapped around a palm tree on the Pacific Coast Highway. Temporary license plate and registration paper-work from the dealership still intact.

TS's kindergarten teacher wondered why he had an Irish Accent. His childhood nanny, Mrs. Doyle, came to pick him up from the hospital that night, just back from visiting her family in Dublin. His parents would have done it, but ya know, it was late, there were still guests at the house, Sheena E had to load out her drum kit, Honey, can you get me another glass of wine . . .

Lifestyles of the rich and _____ (insert your adjective here).

TS had a peacock-colored shell protecting his fragile heart. I was just learning how to use my new wings. They too were peacock-colored. Hey weird, we match. I feel like I know you from somewhere. And that's how these things unfold.

At first it was all excitement, wonder, and quick games of see what's behind-the-shell peak-a-boo. Every time he opened a little, I would scream like a surprised toddler.

I was getting used to my wings. They were heavier than my arms, but could carry me further faster. TS was born with wings, so feigned excitement at watching me learn how to use mine. The dynamic mimicked an excited permit driver, hopping into the sedan of a near-retired drivers' ed teacher. "Whoa, whoa, whoa, not so fast. Brake pedal is the one on the right." (Grumbles) "These friggin' kids . . ."

But when that permit driver skips out of the DMV, brand new license in hand, the anxiously awaiting teacher offers a wide open "You did it!" hug, handing over the coveted sedan keys. Behind his BluBlockers hides a prideful gleam in his eyes. Thata girl!

TS is the first person ever to be able to follow the rapidly bouncing ball of my brain, lighting up when I made a Tolstoy, Tom Waits and Watergate reference in under six syllables. Beyond any logic, the cells in my body would start to clap out the beat to Buddy Holly's "Not Fade Away" anytime they sensed the cells in his body were near. I could feel it in my eyelashes when he walked in the building. I could feel it in my heart when he was thinking about me.

When Chris died, I reviewed all my relationships to date. Writing the "Dear Johns," "Thank You, Davids," and "Do you accept payment plans?" Cleaning It All Up. Important Spiritual Work. In doing so, I reviewed what attracted me to the friends and lovers I chose to keep in my life, and those I was ready to let go of. A workaholic by descent, design and trade, I recognized the thing I most loved in family, friends and friends with benefits, were the ones that:

A. called me out on my shit

B. I could just kick back with in jeans and a tee

After living in LA for so long, I understood why Gwyneth Paltrow wore minimal make-up at her private wedding. It's all just a lot of work after a while.

One person who came to mind as someone I could spend all of eternity with, was my childhood friend EZ-E. We weren't a romantic match, but we had GREAT times together. The kind you know your grandkids will be telling their grandkids about. He lived in my roommate's laundry pile in college, his van in my driveway in Colorado and on my couch in California. Together we could turn life into a carnival wherever we went. Yes, even that one September. Someone had to break the tension every hour or so. Enter *EZ-E* & *me* with stories from the road.

Crazier times consisted of jumping on cross-country flights to avoid regional traffic, calling out of work Monday to catch another couple of Phish Shows, and our personal favorite, driving to the Rock n' Roll Hall of Fame (461.53 miles away) one night, because we couldn't really think of anything else to do. **"You won't do it," Chris would tease us, and then we would of course, go do it.**

I was thinking about how one of my favorite things to do with EZ-E was to watch old Bruce Springsteen Concert DVDs, reciting all the songs, stories and audience screams verbatim from memory, transforming my apartment, his shore house and even the crosstown bus into Madison Square Garden just by pressing "play."

> *"Ya gotta let 'em hear ya in Jersey, man.*
> *Is there anybody really aliiiiiiiiiiiiive out there?"*
>
> —BRUCE SPRINGSTEEN

At that moment, TS texted me he had bought said Box Set and did I want to come over to watch it with him. Please bear in mind we are in Los Angeles, not the Jersey Shore. The pediatricians don't hand out copies of "Born to Run" with your birth certificate here. This was not an isolated coincidence. We were unintentionally in each other's thoughts, dreams and traffic patterns all too often for it to be normal. Like bumping into each other at the Brazilian Barbeque Joint clear on the other side of town in the middle of the workday. We're both vegetarians. I swear I looked around for Cupid and his cunning arrow.

I felt unbelievably connected to TS in a way I had never felt before. He said he felt the same way. I thought to myself, *Hmm, I never thought I would end up with warm-up pants guy, but there it is. These things happen I suppose.*

I talked to EZ-E and his wife, Coco, about it. He assured, "Do you

think Coco wanted to end up with someone like me? No. Helllll no.
You end up with who you are supposed to end up with."

Coco, a buyer for Bergdorf Goodman who sat first row at The Pucci
Show during fashion week each year, smugly rolled her bright purple
MAC makeup-defined eyes at me in unity. Then she kissed EZ-E. He
had the perfect queen for his castle.

Things that make you go "Om."

I was opening up in a brand new way. I liked this softer, quieter version of myself—the version who wasn't in charge of a full staff, a film
set, a famous literary estate and taking down Monsanto. That version of
me was tired. I was finally ready to be taken care of.

So I told TS. (I had never mentioned it to Biggie, as I thought it was
understood.)

TS responded by running around with other women all summer while
my guts were spilled all over the floor. We swam in the same circles, so
I had the pleasure of meeting these new jogging partners of his, week
after week. I wanted to hang myself with their custom-made Adidas
shoelaces. But then thought, *Hey, I used to run a seven-minute mile. Screw
this.* So I did what any publicly mortified, hopped up on coffee, obsessed
with someone who doesn't like her, thirty-something woman would do.
I wrote a painstakingly detailed email that rivaled an F. Scott Fitzgerald
novella—as lovingly undercutting, as cruelly kind. I left no random
thought unexplained. I didn't want to look back on it like I did Biggie,
and wonder what would have happened had I just stayed the four days.
It was a lot. Even for me. However, it was the most honest thing I've
ever said/done in my entire life, so regardless of his response I thought,
I *win. I am participating in life. Chris would be proud.*

TS responded with the following:

*Amy: Life is not a fucking John Hughes movie.
Seriously. Grow up. This is the kind of letter you
send to someone who radically dumped you after 6
months. This isn't the type of thing that you send to
someone who you hung out with a couple of times.*

Heartbroken? How could you be? There was never anything to BE broken from. We are adults. These things happen. Move on.

In my 39 years I've never come across such a distorted sense of reality. Sorry to be so harsh, but really man . . . GET YOUR SHIT TOGETHER, DUDE.

And now we know why he is 39 and single.

Jim Jim Murphy would never talk to a woman (or really, any human being, dog, cat, goldfish, sea monkey) like that. And that's why our moms love him.

This is a great lesson in:

a. When someone tells you who they are, you really should listen. (I know, sometimes it's not so easy to explain that to your heart.)

b. Always take a deep breath, go for a walk or call a friend before pressing send. This guy is likely filing for a restraining order as we speak.

The great news is: Due to a carefully cultivated support system, a deep yoga and meditation practice, and a diet made mostly of awesome veggies from the Organic Farmers' Markets, I did not go off the deep end like I did with Biggie.

Having spent enough of the very precious moments I have on this planet thinking about TS and tripping his jogging partners as they crossed the finish line, I waved the white flag. I surrendered. Their knees were probably bruised by now anyway.

Okay, okay, I let my girlfriends rip him apart for as long as they each liked. However, I did not go into a whole *What If?*—I just went right to my yoga mat. I did some japa meditation practice. I felt the pain fully, wholly, in every corner of my soul, and then . . . I let it pass.

What came to mind was a quote from His Holiness the 14th Dalai Lama of Tibet:

"Remember that not getting what you want is sometimes a wonderful stroke of luck."

HEARTBREAK SYNDROME

"The Truth is everyone is going to hurt you.
You just gotta find the ones worth suffering for."
—BOB MARLEY

Takotsubo cardiomyopathy is a sudden temporary weakening of the muscle around the heart, the myocardium. According to *The New England Journal of Medicine,* Harvard Medical School and Johns Hopkins University Medical School, this condition can be triggered by acute emotional stress such as a break-up or death of a loved one. It is the heart organ's protective measure against a lethal reaction, such as stress cardiomyopathy, which can lead to acute heart failure.

According to the *New England Journal of Medicine,* Takotsubo Cardiomyopathy occurs in four steps:

1. Fear or grief is experienced by the subject.

2. Adrenal glands and nerves react, pumping hormones to handle stress, including adrenaline.

3. The heart can lose its effective pumping ability.

4. Chest pain and/or other heart attack-like symptoms are experienced.

The Heartbreak Yoga Institute of Inquiry clinical prognosis: That bricks-on-chest and/or punched-in-the-stomach feeling is legit. The guys in the white coats concur.

Julie Kokesch, M.A.—PSB 36597, Psychological Assistant, Counseling Center of Santa Monica

Amy: Jules, you're a psychologist, what is the diagnosis for someone who has totally lost their minds in love?

Julie: When people fall in love, many chemicals in the brain get activated. The new brain activity is usually seen in the areas of "instinct" and "euphoria." The beginnings of this process are when we usually feel infatuated with the other person and that is when our brain is literally cascading with new chemicals. This cascade actually overrides the brains ability for "logic" and "reason." This can look like running to Vegas to get married in the first two weeks of dating and moving in together in the first month of meeting. The logical and reasoning part of the brain is less accessible when the cascade is flowing. The other term we've often used is "Punch Drunk Love" which is partially from the term "Punch Drunk," which is a boxing term for when a boxer gets hit too hard in the head and tweety birds are circling his head. Adding the word "Love" to Punch Drunk is a cute mockery of how a friend who is in love may appear to be behaving. Do not make any major life decisions while in this stage. Yes, it's fun—enjoy it, but understand you are under the influence of some powerful chemicals in your brain.

In the beginning/infatuated phase, it's all about the neurochemistry: dopamine, norepinephrine and serotonin are more responsible for the attraction part of the relationship. The effects on the brain look strangely similar to the same effects of obsessive-compulsive disorder, or at least temporarily. A testosterone increase also leads to increased sexual attraction and sexual behavior. Later in a relationship, oxytocin and vasopressin are responsible for long-term bonding and attachment. Nerve growth factor levels can increase and stay increased for up to a year before they come back down to normal level. Another effect these chemicals can do to the brain is cause you to lose your appetite as well as lose sleep, so be prepared to be skinny, tired, horny and happy.

Amy: What is the clinical diagnosis for someone who is crashing from the love high? Or worse, gets kicked to the curb?

Julie: Well, on the flip side, when all of these chemicals have gone back to their normal levels and the love interest is still around, this is the "falling" part of falling in love.

The problem with some people is that these chemical reactions that occur at the beginning of all relationships can mimic that of a drug high. Some people can attempt to become addicted to these brain-produced drugs and the result is usually disappointing. People do not realize that it's a normal process and it is not a constant state of being. That is why I say to enjoy every second of it because that is how the system was intended to work. The caution is in the expectation that the high of "falling" in love will remain a constant. That's almost as unrealistic as expecting to stay drunk for thirty days straight after one night out of partying.

Opening your heart to a deeper love and opening your mind to a deeper respect of yourself and someday your partner . . . yes, for some this is where the vulnerability is increased and may seem a little scary. But if you dare to "go there," then the rewards are well worth it. In my opinion, label relationships as work, but I challenge you to re-label the experience of relationships as fun.

Amy: Challenge Accepted.

Shiva Rea—Exhale Center for Sacred Movement

We are all born lovers with the natural instinct to bond and love. The very nature of our heart cells are to syncopate, to bond in rhythm. Our first heartbeat begins in the womb spontaneously without a signal from the brain. Some 10,000 pacemaker cells begin in unison.

This rhythm of these specialized heart cells also creates an energetic charge that creates the strongest energy field of any part of the body that radiates outward at least 10 feet away, like an inner sun with the capacity to communicate with other "heart fields" as well as perceive the energetic field that envelops the earth and reflects the same qualities of dissonant and coherence—being in synch or out of synch with the world around us.

We can feel this energetic heat within our body when we place our hand upon another person's back—this is our heartfire—"el Corazon de

Fuego," "Cid agni," Leve" as envisioned and invoked by the world's ancestral traditions and throughout western culture. The heart's "fire" is both a literal part of the organ's energetic heat but also the love, passion, wisdom, intelligence, intuitive knowing, presence of being fully alive qualities universally assigned to our heart.

Love is the healing wisdom that is our very cellular nature of our heart. Love is even the gravitational attraction that keeps us bonded to our earth mother in the infinite space. Love is the rasa of yoga—the transforming nectar of the heart released through the fire of one's practice and life churnings in passion and in grief, in tenderness and in inherent peace. Aham Prema—our very nature is love.

GRACE

"Don't chase boys. Chase grace."

—SRIDHAR SILBERFEIN, THE CENTER FOR SPIRITUAL STUDIES

After the Biggie debacle, before my direct deposit hit, I used my surfboard as a couch, dining room table and even guest bed. I lived in Venice Beach at The Breakwater, Westside LA's sweetest surf spot. I would stick my sleepy head out the window many mornings to give the surf report by cell: "Mushy." "Crumbly." "Close Out." "Offshore winds, with three feet lefts—get over here!"

I made a great friend named Shima. She and I spent many a Sunday afternoon studying the waves, but more pointedly, the boys that rode them. Ripped guys in wetsuits would catch "glassies." Shima and I would try to catch them.

Quick thinking, fast-talking, go get 'em, New York City-bred Film Production Girls, we went after the waves (and the boys) like we did everything else—hard, fast, and with a defined attainable goal. Our objective was twofold:

1. Learn how to surf

2. Learn how to surf with cute surfer boys

We would paddle out into the "lineup" and wait with everyone else for the next "swell." As the waves peaked prior to the horizon the surfers in synchronicity would segue from the vertical ocean observation posture to belly down on the board facing shore. To catch a wave you paddle in the exact right direction, at the exact right speed for that wave. You must position your body weight evenly on the board so the nose doesn't dip, flipping you over. If your legs are too tense, rigid, uneven or floppy, you will likely "pearl" the board and get sucked under. There are so many conditions that have to be exactly right. However, if all the elements align and that wave scoops you up, holds you in its hand, and you let go long enough to "pop up," you can likely stand on the board and coast into shore. During this process you are so totally awake and aware of each micro-movement—the wave, the wind, the board, your body—there is no high like it. What's missing in this equation is the mind. There is no thinking in surfing. There is only feeling and doing. Mostly the doing gets done by trying not to do too much. You can't "think" your way into surfing. Either you catch a wave or you don't. The conditions are either right, or they're not. End of story.

Often the *old schoolers* would advise us *kooks,* "That looks like a good wave for you, see how it is rolling slow? Why don't you try for that one?"

But not us—hard, fast, and thinking we can do it all on our own, Shima and I would race into the lineup and "go for" the hardest, fastest, highest wave. Hard and fast + Hard and fast does not equal a smooth ride. When our egos would ripen and we would "think" we had it all figured out, Mother Ocean in all her glory would crash over us, pull us under, thrash us around, and catapult us to shore—*if* we were lucky. There were plenty of times I was knocked in the head so hard with the board or beaten into the beach bottom with such force that I thought I might never surface, or survive.

Gasping for air, not sure where the wave broke, where my board was, where Shima was, where the shore was, where I was, I would gain my bearings and get back out there—stronger than the set before.

A few years after The Great Engagement Party Massacre, I bumped into Biggie at a mutual friend's wedding in New Jersey. Let's be honest—I worked out for three months, got my roots dyed, a fresh mani-pedi and flew 3,000 miles knowing I would "bump" into Biggie at our mutual friend's wedding.

The usual scene ensued. To recap:

We would see each other.

Our eyes would light up.

We would run toward each other like a soap opera montage, get all excited talking fast with our hands about nothing at all, touching each other every chance we got—and then when the pacing slowed and we stared deep into each other's eyes, about to admit something life altering, some girl who made it to the final qualifying round at the Playboy Mansion but was only hired as an alternate would put her perfectly manicured hand around his waist, signifying ownership. At which point he and I would ease into a conversation about the weather or whatever.

This time however, there was no ease, or talk of unseasonable heat. The storm was already brewing. When the Miss Teen USA-type, two sizes too big for her JC Penny junior prom dress, tried the territorial pissing waist-grab move, I just stood there and stared. All those hours watching "The Dog Whisperer" really paid off. Shima regarded Cesar Milan as a dating coach more than a dog trainer. In that moment, I proved to be pack leader. Like everything else, I came there hard and fast with a defined attainable goal—to find out what happened to him that night and why I wasn't Little Mrs. Biggie. The conversation went like this:

Biggie: You look good.

I wonder how much she hates me?

Amy: I know.

I better. I spent three months preparing for this!

Biggie: How is Cali?

Are you going to live there forever or is there still a chance with us? And also, do I have a chance to sleep with you tonight?

Amy: Great.

I have a great career, great friends, great apartment and a great yoga practice, but I still think about you . . . a lot.

Biggie: Yeah?

So . . . are you always going to live there, or are you going to move back here and move in with me? Think I can sleep with you tonight?

Amy: Yeah.

Yes, it's awesome, but yes, I would live with you if you would just ask, you idiot.

Biggie: You think you'll always live there?

So . . . do I still have a chance, or do you completely hate me. You know I'm working for my dad now, right? I had to sell the condo. So, if you sleep with me tonight, I'll have to get a hotel room. My apartment is pathetic. Should I get a hotel room?

Amy: For the foreseeable future, yes. I really love it. I mean, unless I had a reason to be somewhere else.

I love it, but I love you more. I don't care about your job or your home. Put a ring on it already!

Biggie: Unless you had a reason, huh?

So . . . you don't hate me and you might sleep with me tonight?

Amy: What the hell happened to you that night?

Biggie: What night?

Amy: (I stared at him Cesar Milan-style. Calm. Assertive.)

Biggie: (*Starting to panic*) I called you but I couldn't leave a message. Your phone was off but the voicemail was full. By the time the guys left I thought it was too late. I called but I didn't get a hold of you. I . . . I . . . I . . .

Amy: So?!

You aren't going to get off on a technicality. Why did you change your mind? Why didn't you keep your word? Is something wrong with me? I thought you liked me.

Biggie: So?!

I don't knooooow. I screwed up. Yes I liked you.

Amy: You said you were going to show and you just NEVER showed up.

How could you do that to me?

Biggie: I know but I called you.

I know I screwed up. I was scared.

Amy: I never talked to you or got a message, or a follow-up message or phone call or email or MySpace message or text message or a carrier pigeon.

Scared?! So was I, but I didn't humiliate you in front of your best friend's entire 46-person family!

Biggie: What did you care? You didn't like me anyway—you were off in [imitates surfers] Cali Bro.

I didn't know if I was good enough for you.

Amy: Well, I wasn't [imitates Biggie imitating surfers] "Off in Cali Bro" when I was stood up at Sue's engagement party.

Mortified. Heartbroken. Wondering where you were, you asshole.

Biggie: You didn't need me there. You can do everything on your own. Look at you. Look at everything that you have done. What did you need me for?

I didn't know you wanted me there so bad. I thought you didn't care. What do you want me to do about it now?

Amy: Yeah, but I wanted you there. I mean, I wanted you.

I know I can, but it doesn't mean I always want to. I loved you. You really hurt me.

Biggie: You did?

You mean I am good enough for you? You do like me? And you WILL sleep with me?

Amy: Yeah, I did.

As the words came out of my mouth, I realized how much they rang true. "I did." Meaning, I don't now. Past tense. Wow. I had mentally compartmentalized this whole Biggie Breakdown Business as "Present Tense" for so long. Even when one of the buff surfers took me on a "date" (read a bike ride, beer and burrito), I compared him to Biggie the whole time, as though he were some perfect benchmark to be basing everything off of. This real-life Biggie didn't come anywhere close to the Clark Gable, Kelly Slater, Dave Grohl-guy that was running around my head playing finders keepers losers weepers with my heart.

I mean, he's a fine human I'm honored to have been emotionally annihilated by—he loves God, his country, George W. Bush, deer hunting and the NRA, but is that a lifelong teammate match for my hippie ass? Not so sure.

As this realization wrapped around me in real time, he finally said the words I had been hoping to hear for years. The words I had been longing for and fantasizing about while I walked the red carpet of my first feature film premiere at Ziegfeld's Theatre in New York City; while I sat among the nominees, fourth row, at The Academy Awards watching Katherine Bigelow make history; while I had a meeting in the famed boardroom of super agency CAA overlooking The Hollywood Sign; while I whined about it to "_____" and "The_____" at a Christmas Party; while my friends Jamie and Diana assured me I was good enough "as is"; while Jonathan Rhys Meyers said, "You're gorgeous dahling, forget the cheeky maggot" and Alex O'Lachlan echoed, "Dewhurst, get over the bastard"; while my cousin Jen rolled her eyes, "Are we still talking about this? He's an ass"; while my friends Rob and

Gaby set me up with everyone they knew; while I chatted with George Clooney at the Hotel Bel Air; while my friend Kim dragged me ice skating; while my friends Kadi & Shima politely pretended to listen as they secretly watched *The Dog Whisperer;* on the other end of the phone, while Ali, Sue, Jim Jim Murphy and the hen house told me I was too good for him; and just before I threw my surfboard in the water at The Breakwater the previous weekend. Yes. I heard the words I had longed to hear:

"You know I've always loved you."

VICTORY!!! (Or, as my people say in Sanskrit *Hanuman Ki Jai.*)

Mom, book the church. Sue, call the caterer. Ali, order the dress. Virgin Galactic, I need two first class tickets to the moon, all my dreams are coming true. Wahoooo!

"I just figured when I was ready to settle down you would move back home with me. You've always been 'the one' you know that."

Ahh, I've always been "The One." I did know that.

Wait a second, hold on. In the words of the great Foghorn Leghorn "Hamana, Hamana, I said, I said . . . " When HE was ready?! When HEEEEEEEE was ready?! So let me get this straight. I'm in the first generation of women to challenge approximately 200,000 years of biology, fully expected to have a fulltime job, nurture it into a career, work just as hard if not harder than the boys (mentally AND physically), build and care for a home, go out with the girls for so-and-so's birthday, make it to wedding showers, baby showers, christenings, first birthday parties with a present in my hand. Still put something in savings each month. Keep up on current affairs, the death toll in Iraq and Afghanistan, the national debt and what Suri Cruise is wearing that week. Download the latest software for my iPhone and figure out where all the f-ing buttons are now, pay my bills on time, know what big-businesses are and are not putting GMOs in our foods, remember to bring that 20% off coupon to Bed, Bath and Beyond, get my oil changed every 3,000 miles, make my next day's lunch with the allotted fat, protein, carbohydrate ratio and calorie count, brush, floss and say my prayers before bed, being sure to hit the treadmill, the tennis court, or the yoga mat somewhere in there so I look decent doing it all. I've somehow managed to pull ALL of this off by myself (high five Wonder Woman), and now *HE* decides when/ where/how *I* settle down? How *MY* life unfolds?

I'm calling Gloria Steinem. This is bullshit.

How had I unconsciously given away all this time, energy, personal power, prana and maha amazing moments? WHAT was I thinking? I remember wailing to Sue, "How could he have done this to me?" Now I was mentally wailing, *How could I have done this to myself?* It hadn't occurred to me how much of my life I had thrown out by having my head somewhere else, somewhere far away, with someone who didn't deserve it. I wasn't fully present during any of the aforementioned moments. I was pining for something outside myself—something I thought would "make it all better." It hadn't occurred to me that *I* was the one who could make it all better. Now *I* was the one playing finders keepers with my heart, and I wasn't going to be so careless in the next round. Bhaja Govinda.

As I was planning my exit strategy and figuring out how to get a hold of Ani DiFranco, Miss *Busted* USA came back over to bother us, yapping like a hungry Chihuahua "Christaphhhaaaaa." This time I let her lead the pack. I had waves to catch back at The Breakwater.

After an *Endless Summer* at Sunday afternoon "Surf Camp," Shima and I now understood why surfers are always portrayed as stoners. A day in the sun and surf, getting bounced between your board and the sandy bottom of the Breakwater, really can beat you up. Suddenly the beer, bong rip, burrito cure-all doesn't seem so strange.

One evening during the sunset swell, I was whiney because I hadn't caught the last wave. Shima was whiney because she hadn't caught the last boy. A no-nonsense girl (with low blood sugar, and a bruised bum from getting bounced around) she snapped: "It wasn't your wave."

I snapped back: "He wasn't your boy."

Shima: "There's always another boy."

Amy: "And there's always another wave. Hey . . . you tricked me. That was your line."

We laughed, hopped on our bikes, grabbed a burrito and rode the bike path, flirting with surf and skate boarders we rode past, "Caaaaatch Aaaaanything?"

Biggie called me two summers ago.

He had just bought a fixer-upper down the block from his folks, and was wondering when I would be in town to visit. It had been a few years, and he was "just wondering" how I was.

I had just returned from Rome, Italy, where Ali and I took Kim to see Bruce Springsteen for her 35th birthday. We sang "Surprise, Surprise" so loud, they probably *did* hear us in Jersey. I was doing laundry and repacking for next weekend's trip to France where I would be location scouting for a feature film about *Feast*ing in Paris.

I was impressed by his safety, security and stability.

He was impressed by my life of adventure.

Opposites still attract.

We nestled into the same ol' conversation; talking excitedly about the details of those differences, how the yapping Chihuahua was now peeing on some other guy's leg, highlights from Sue and Jim Jim Murphy's Wedding, the big Halloween Party, that one September, and sparring political points of view. I have to give it to him—somehow, after all this time, I still caught myself swooning as he made well-educated points about public policy sound sexy. I could see those big browns sparkling, even on a bad cell connection. However, as the conversation slowed and it turned into the ever so loaded, "So, you still like it out there?" section, I caught myself just answering, "Yup," without the heavy subtext. Just, "Yup."

Everything was lighter now. Everything just flowed with ease. There wasn't a pushing and pulling, tugging and breaking, thinking and doing, planning and executing. My life was unfolding as intended—gratefully flowing in the "Wave of Grace."

One of my most revered teachers, Krishna Das, opens his events with a version of the following:

> *"We're going to start with a short prayer. It's a prayer of Grace. Grace is what wakes us up when we're asleep. Grace is what removes obstacles from our path. Obstacles we don't even know are there. Grace is what arranges our lives. So we're forced to look within, and if you're anything like me, you haaave to be forced. And if you're here now, it's because grace is operating inside of your life flow . . ."*

I'm sure you've heard the hymn *Amazing Grace.* As a kid, you don't really get why old ladies of the church choir would cluck something like this so passionately. *Ewww, did she say wretch or roach?* As an adult you start to understand its content. The practices of yoga, meditation, mantra and kirtan were like luminary Lasik Surgery for me. In other words, "I once was blind, but now I see."

Seventeen years of dead cell batteries, has-been playboy bunnies, miscommunications, missed flights, missed moments. Nothing about Biggie and me was ever in this "Wave of Grace." None of the elements ever aligned. Okay, once—ONE weekend when I was paddling at the exact right speed, at the exact right time.

Biggie wasn't my wave.

Grace was operating in the divine design that time by pulling me under, thrashing me around and cracking me WIDE OPEN. If I weren't all alone on a strange beach, in a strange city, in a strange swell, underwater, gasping for air, I may not have grabbed on to these practices with such fervor. I may not have studied like my life depended on it, because as it turns out it did. It does. Just when I thought I was going to drown, Sara Ivanhoe threw me a life raft (or a yoga mat, as the case may be).

Everyone Has a Biggie

Be it a near-miss puppy love never meant to be, an orgasmic lover, or longtime life partner, the experience of loss is tangible. It could be a job, a home, or an industry that in the internet age just kinda went away. It could be the future you had hoped for little John-o or the next 70 years you had planned with your husband. It could be the promotion or award, the trajectory you had worked toward and somehow missed. The stability. The adventure. Life is filled with a million little heartbreaks. But if we don't get out there and in the game, what's even the point of living? In about a hundred years we'll all be gone and none of the humiliations and half-completed to-do lists will have mattered. The only thing that will have mattered is how you treated yourself, your loved ones, and this awe-inspiring moment.

"You won't do it" Chris would say, and then we would of course, go do it.

There's this wondrous alchemy in the moments when you are so raw, when you have no fight left in you, no walls to protect. The exposed beautiful, awful, wonderful, terrible, gorgeous being with all your humor and faults and perceived rights and wrongs shines through. This is a humbling, but powerful place to be, because you can connect to the real you. The radiant being who isn't associated with names, job titles, zip codes, tax brackets, social circles, romantic relationships, wave classifications, shoe choices. All the things we define ourselves by. When it is just the raw you, the blood and the guts and the tears and the thorns, you are in an extraordinary position. You are at the bottom. "Hollow bone" the Native Americans call it.

Empty.

From here you can be anything.

There is nothing in the cup.

You choose what to fill it back up with.

Mother Teresa once said, "I know God will not give me anything I can't handle. I just wish he didn't trust me so much." I'm not imposing a happy ending, or a deus ex machina moment, I am however extending my belief that Grace (God, Jesus, Allah, Muhammad, Buddha, Ammachi, Maharaj-ji, Jah, the Universe) would not have given you this if you were unable to handle it. *You are stronger then you think.*

Oh, and Shima did go out with the surfer who bailed on her. Home by 7:30 she said, "I'm glad I went out with him. I now know in a beer and a half exactly how much energy to expend on another human being."

TS wasn't my wave either. I didn't need a beer and a half to figure that out. Grace (disguised as a gnarly email) did it for me.

"You go up, you go down, you go up you go down.
It's all grace. Just breathe."

—SRIDHAR SILBERFEIN, THE CENTER FOR SPIRITUAL STUDIES

"It's Alright Ma, I'm Only Bleeding."
—BOB DYLAN

Priestess Laura Ambika Lalita Amazzone—Author, Teacher, Jewelry Artist, and Yogini

"In my experience, the greater the heartbreak, the more I recognize how much I have allowed my heart to open and love. The beauty is, once we have loved with an open, trusting, expanded heart, once we have surrendered to the grace of Love's mysteries, there is really no going back to that smaller space our heart inhabited before we fell in love. We are forever changed in the union, in the separation, and especially in feeling how Love, in its paradoxical blessings of pleasure and pain, is ultimately an invitation to love ourselves more fully."

Varun Soni

Varun Soni is the Dean of Religious Life at the University of Southern California. He received his B.A. degree in Religion from Tufts University, where he also earned an Asian Studies minor and completed the program in Peace and Justice Studies. He subsequently received his M.T.S. degree from Harvard Divinity School and his M.A. degree through the Department of Religious Studies at UCSB. He went on to receive his J.D. degree from UCLA School of Law, where he also completed the Critical Race Studies Program and served as the Chief Articles Editor for UCLA's Journal of Islamic and Near Eastern Law. He earned his Ph.D. through the Department of Religious Studies at the University of Cape Town, where his doctoral research focused on religion and popular culture. As an undergraduate student, Dean Soni spent a semester living in a Buddhist monastery in Bodh Gaya, India, through Antioch University's Buddhist Studies Program. As a graduate student, he spent months doing field research in South Asia through UCSB's Center for Sikh and Punjab Studies.

Varun is currently a University Fellow at USC Annenberg's Center on Public Diplomacy. He is a member of the State Bar of California, the American Academy of Religion, and the Association for College and University Religious Affairs. He is on the advisory board for the Center for Muslim-Jewish Engagement, the Music Preservation Project, Cross-Currents, and the Journal for Interreligious Dialogue.

Amy: Why do you think we get our asses totally kicked sometimes?

Dean Soni: From the perspective of Indian Religions, the dharma religions—Hinduism, Buddhism, Jainism, Sikhism, real spiritual development, revolution and development occurs when you understand the true nature of yourself and that means that you have to go beyond ego. So what happens when you get knocked down or beat up, or thrown on the ground is that many of your conceptions of self that you think, your ideas of who you are, your own self of identity get shaken, to the core.

From an Indian Spiritual Perspective, that's good because it shakes you out of an ego-driven existence. You may think that you are this or you are that, but when things don't go your way, that really challenges that conception of ego. So, from a spiritual perspective, that's where real growth can occur; when you are outside of your comfort zone. Throughout history we see many religious leaders who have this experience of being knocked down—getting their ego put in check and then awakening to some greater realization.

There's a great saying in India: "The fruit takes a long time to ripen, but it falls in a single moment." So a fruit on a tree can take a long time to get ripe but the moment it falls, it can be at any moment and it happens instantaneously. So too, can our experience of enlightenment, of awakening. We're not sure when that moment may happen. It may take a long time to ripen, and in the Indian tradition, I think it's more likely that that moment will happen at a time when your ego has been challenged, or deconstructed, sort of destroyed completely and you have to rebuild a sense of self from the ground up. I'm sure every religious guru has had this experience.

One such example is Mahatma Gandhi.

The reason why Gandhi became a great spiritual leader who focused on social justice is because he had a pretty traumatic experience when he was a young lawyer in South Africa. He trained as a lawyer in England, then went to South Africa. He had a first-class ticket on a train from Pretoria. He was Indian, and at that time in South Africa, Indians couldn't sit in first class. There was a legalized racial segregation. He got thrown off the train because he refused to move. That awakened him to the plight of others. Before that, he was a well-educated, elite, privileged lawyer who felt that "Because I'm a lawyer, I should have all these kinds of privileges and I should be held in high esteem." When he was thrown off the train, it made him empathetic to what all Indians were going through. Had he not had that experience, had his ego not been checked, had he not been put in a place where he had to reevaluate who he was and what he actually deserved, I don't think he would have become the Mahatma. He tells of this powerful experience in his autobiography. It really made him empathetic and compassionate to the suffering of others—others who were victims of racial segregation. And so he pioneered to South Africa, and the rest is history.

So, one of the things I think getting knocked down does, or having your ego challenged does, is that in your own suffering you become more empathetic or compassionate to the suffering of others. That cultivates a real sense of self. In the Indian tradition the real "I" is not born, it does not die, it exists over time; and who I am and who you are, are not two different things. When we understand that, when we get beyond the personal ego, then we understand the self is a type of universal self—a universal consciousness, and that's where the real spiritual growth happens.

> *"Without struggle, there is no progress."*
> —FREDERICK DOUGLAS

Dr. Dianna Wuagneux

Dr. Dianna Wuagneux provides on-call advisement to the US Department of Defense with a focus on Nations in Transition/Fragile States including, Central Asia, Middle East, North Africa, Former Soviet Union.

She has served as a Peace & Development Advisor for the UNDP, focused on issues of border stabilization and reconciliation, both internal and regional (Uzbekistan, Kyrgyzstan, Afghanistan, Tajikistan, China).

Dr. Wuagneux worked as the Executive Advisor Reconciliation & Reconstruction for the U.S. Department of Defense JIEDDO, XVIII Airborne Corps in Iraq. In this position, she provided expertise as executive advisor relevant to Conflict Resolution, Disarmament, Demobilization and Reintegration, improving quality of life via conflict mitigation, COIN, nation-building, cross-border negotiations, governance, civil-society, capacity building, reconstruction and development

to the General Officers, and senior members of the staff under their com-
mand. As part of this role, she designated and prioritized projects, programs and activities, including but not limited to: education, healthcare
(immunization programs, building/equipping of community health clin-
ics and hospitals, participation in physician/nurse/midwife recruiting and
training efforts, etc.) markets, roads, utilities, government services, and
small business assistance.

She has a seat on the United Nations "Permanent Forum for Indige-
nous Issues," has been awarded the NATO Medal for her service to the
International Security Assistance Force, and has been called upon to provide written opinions to Congress and the DOD regarding the surge in
Iraq, as well as interagency (DOS/DOD) relations in North Africa and
the Middle East.

She is published in journals such as Leverage, the Systems' Thinker,
and Cultural Survival Quarterly. She is regularly interviewed as an
"expert" in behavioral economics in newspapers/periodicals, and is frequently asked to address field practitioners, academics, and assorted pol-
icymakers at international conferences and symposia.

This smart, strong, beautiful and brave woman has always been one
of my heroes. She has the innate ability to handle unimaginable conflict
and crisis on a global scale, and yet stay open-hearted, kind, and compassionate. I asked Dr. Wuagneux about rites of passage, dating rituals,
heartbreak, grief, grace, pain and spiritual awakening around the world.
From an undisclosed off-grid location, she kindly responded via dial-up
internet:

Very deep thinking. I see you are becoming quite the philosopher.
Good for you! Now, to your question . . .

Rites of passage are, by their nature those events that leave us
changed. We see less violence/anti-social behavior among young men
raised in culture where rites of passage are formalized. Here in the
modern West, many young men (and women) spend years trying to
figure out when they are "grown-up," and what that means. An
insightful quote by Michael Meade states, "What initiates us also strips

us down to the inner essentials and releases qualities and powers that were hidden within."

Grief/heartbreak does that to us. Some do not recover, but even those who do, are changed. All cultures see these events forms of passage. It changes our place in society. Is a person married, widowed, separated, or divorced? We see these states differently from one another, and treat people accordingly; e.g., if a woman is engaged to a soldier and he is killed, is she treated as a widow? Is a person still seen as a parent, even if their child(ren) has/have died? In my case, I am no longer anyone's daughter; in the blink of an eye, I went from being just one of many in an extended family, to the family matriarch. My role has changed. This has forced me to see myself differently and figure out how these differences will be expressed by me and what I might expect from others toward me. Big doings. More enjoyably, I think about what good I gained from knowing my mother and being her daughter, and how can I use this good in a way that allows me to grow from it and share it with others.

When I worked in the Middle East, Central Asia, & India, etc., my colleagues were mortified when I told them about my three children and their on-going dating sagas. Their daughters would not be out with a boy until that boy had been chosen to be a new son-in-law. They could not understand why we would allow our youth to go through so much pain. In our society, most adults will say that these earlier heartbreaks are so painful that they help prepare young people for pains to come. **I think our culture does a disservice in painting a picture that leads us to believe that if we are in pain, then we have done something wrong. Pain is part of life.**

As for the ass-kickings (well said, by the way), I believe the answer is connected to the issue above. We experience and endure heartbreak because we are alive and we care. Those who don't care are dangerous, (we call them psycho/sociopaths) and it is wise to steer clear of them. Most of the time, when we get hit with the wrecking-ball-of-life, it is because we went ahead with something/someone when we already knew better. But the lure of excitement over stability, the mysterious over the staid, or the possibility over the rut can be nearly impossible to resist. And usually, once we recover from the blow, we look back and still say it was worth it. The alternative to life with pain, is to be inert. Pain is how we grow—a self-correcting mechanism if you will, and some people have greater tolerance for it than others. Many of them become the adventurers, leaders, and heroes through time.

Now the other kind of pain—the out-of-the-blue type (unexpected death of a loved one, sudden and unexpected physical or emotional trauma caused by accident or injury), for example happens because while we are busy focusing on our life, the lives of others are intertwined and once in a while, intersect with violence, i.e. the drunk driver that maims, the bomber/shooter who wraps others into his delusion, the psychological issues of a friend or partner that leads to emotional scars. Most people never feel that this kind of pain was worthwhile. Although, in some belief systems, the pain would be accepted as their dharma, and that it had been planned with the cooperation of other souls before birth. These individuals use this belief to cope.

Your question about the revelation of one's path/dharma as a result of suffering does well to complete the circle. In other words, if one stays in suffering/anger, one does not grow. They stay stuck. In order to get past the suffering, one comes to understand the hurt to be part of an *event*. The way of life is to experience events that change us and incorporate what has been learned into our newly forged selves. How do we know what we learned? We can't until the initial fear/anger resulting from separation begins to pass. Then we can begin to ask ourselves gentle questions about what has changed, and what remains the same. From there, we can figure out what we have to work with for the present. As far as "why" goes, that is where strict religious upbringing can help. Some of the people I have met with total peace of mind live in some of the harshest circumstances on the Earth— think Somalia or Yemen. They suffer less because they firmly believe that Allah pulls all of the strings, and knows what he's doing. Why worry? If only the rest of us could deal so easily with "why." I do think that it is best answered with the passage of time. It is amazing how much sense our lives seem to make when we view our past over our shoulders—when the rhythm and patterns become visible.

Thank you for your good wishes. As for my current transition, I cannot shake the feeling that my mother is wonderfully happy, and that helps. And, being the matriarch? So far, it is great fun.

Christopher Key Chapple, Ph.D.

Christopher Key Chapple, Ph.D., is the Navin and Pratima Doshi Professor of Indic and Comparative Theology at Loyola Marymount University. Dr. Chapple received his undergraduate degree in Comparative Literature and Religious Studies from the State University of New York at Stony Brook and his doctorate in the History of Religions through the Theology Department at Fordham University. He served as Assistant Director of the Institute for Advanced Studies of World Religions and taught Sanskrit, Hinduism, Jainism, and Buddhism for five years at the State University of New York at Stony Brook before joining the faculty at LMU.

Dr. Chapple's research interests have focused on the renouncer religious traditions of India: Yoga, Jainism, and Buddhism. He has published several books, including *Karma and Creativity* (1986), a co-translation of the *Yoga Sutras* of Patanjali (1991), *Nonviolence to Animals, Earth, and Self in Asian Traditions* (1993), *Hinduism and Ecology* (2000), a co-edited volume, *Jainism and Ecology: Nonviolence in the Web of Life* (2002), and *Reconciling Yogas* (2003).

Amy: I've been told that in the great romantic love story of the Bhagavad Gita, The Gopi Gita, the ballad of Radha and Krishna embodies the many aspects of love—excitement, love/romance/lust, separation anxiety knowing they will have to leave one another, the pain felt from that separation and then finally feeling whole or together even when separate. Can you break it down for me?

Chris Chapple: There are so many different levels to heartbreak and love, but there is, of course, the anticipation and the courtship, which is the pursuit, and this is both descriptive of what human beings go through, but is also metaphorical about the spiritual quest. Because in the beginning, what is it that prompts us as we were reading the Chandogya Upanishads today; it's this yearning, it's this hunger, it's this desire, and this being in a place of—we might even call it death, before we manifest into our true selves. Out of that we get a yearning, we get a hankering, we begin to set our intentions on a particular goal.

Now, in terms of courtship, it means that we are in pursuit of a person, but in terms of spiritual life, it means that we have felt an aloneness within ourselves that can't be filled. It can't be filled by things or people, and we then come into a desire to have a spiritual orientation. With relationship, in my instance, [I] got married. You know—the courtship led to marriage, which has been a state of enduring happiness. With faith, or with a spiritual life, there is a feeling of relief and certainty; of being held by having a relationship with something greater than ourselves. In the instance of a Hare Krishna Devotee, it could be devotion to Lord Krishna; in the instance of Christian, it could be devotion to Christ; for a Shaivaite, fashioning one's life around Lord Shiva. And that relationship requires, whether it is a spiritual relationship or a marriage relationship, it requires constant tending and in that constant tending there is remembrance. There are bids to the wife to stay in relationship and of course communication. My parents, as well as her parents, had very, very, very long marriages, 'til death parted them. What we watched with both is that they communicated. My parents would come home. They would sit in the car. They would talk. They were never really without a constant exchange. Exchange of information. An exchange of intimacy. And like that, with spiritual life you have to converge, you have to communicate, you have to align, you have to practice—with a yoga practice, an asana practice. It's really a form of sustained prayer, and with the performance of asana there's a reconnection to that. It could be nameable, but usually it's unnamable. That feeling of Shraddha. The foundation of faith.

> *"Love is a consistent passion to give,*
> *not a meek persistent hope to receive."*
> —Lord Krishna

PART III

Yoga

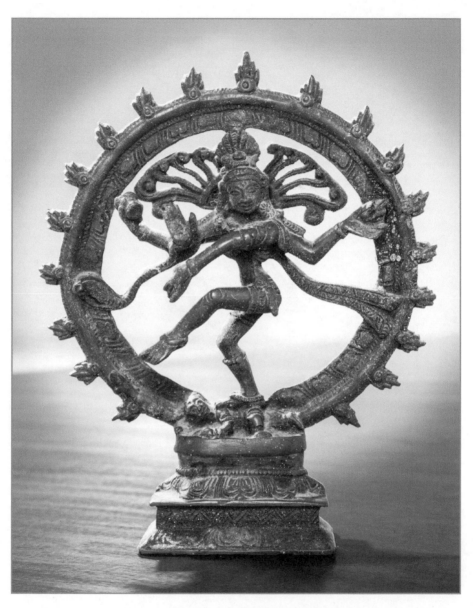

"Dancing Nataraj" by David Young-Wolff

YogaWorks • Main Street, Santa Monica, CA

CHAPTER 6

Sara

"My Foolish Heart (Bhaja Govinda)."

—Krishna Das

Sara Ivanhoe knocked on the door of my heart.

I ducked from view, hoping she wouldn't see I was home.

She knocked again.

And again.

And yet again.

She just wouldn't go away.

She can be so annoying sometimes.

Sara is a master yoga teacher, scholar, and sadhu. She is also one of my best friends. For many years I worked part time as her assistant, apprentice, and eventually took over the business side of her empire, Yoganation. During this time I watched literally thousands of people at classes, workshops, conferences and festivals come up to her after a class, crying and unraveling about how she saved their lives.

"Your Russell Simmons DVD was the first time I did yoga."

"When you taught Jeff Conway to walk on Celebrity Rehab, my whole family was crying!"

"That holistic doctor you sent me to alleviated all my pain."

"That agent you introduced me to got me my dream role."

"Thank you for teaching me to be sexy again after the baby."

"You saved my marriage."

"Sara is the one who introduced us! Sweetie, come here and say thank you to Sara."

She had the great honor of officiating one of these students' weddings—one of the happiest, proudest moments of her life.

Between sweat-inducing vinyasas, some of the usual yogis flowed in . . .

"Sara helps us peel off all the layers of distracting stuff with breath and movement, and then suggests we ask the question: "Is there anything the Universe wants me to know?' I get answers in there because I become quiet and still enough to listen. I wish I could meditate and do that any time I want—but for now, I'll keep going to Sara's class."
—Kristina Brittenham, Lawyer, Pacific Palisades, CA

"I find Sara an incredibly challenging, smart and spiritual teacher. She has great sequencing and mixes it up so every class feels fresh. I always leave feeling energized and calm."
—Deb Schoeneman, Writer/HBO's *Girls*

"Challenging, enriching, heart-pumping, but most of all a blast, Sara Ivanhoe never disappoints while leading the best 90 minutes of yoga in LA."
—Joshua Levine, Novelist/ *Shangrila*, Topanga, CA

"Sara's classes are like Grateful Dead concerts; no two are ever the same. I love Sara's energy and passion when it comes to all things Yoga. She's a gifted teacher who isn't timid about exploring new avenues on the road to spiritual enlightenment, both hers and her students."
—Billy Gottlieb, Music Supervisor, Hollywood Hills, CA

"Sara is a straight up guru. I've been practicing with her for four years and I hope to continue this privileged journey for the rest of my life. Why? Because her yoga never stops oper 'ng my body and mind."
—Matthew Lifschultz, Produce; Westside LA

"As I rarely get a chance to catch a breather in life, one tends to forget what is important. Sara reminds me to not take everything so seriously as she mentally takes us to an internal place. Physically, her efforts to perfect alignment instill discipline while I'm given the challenge. I'm grateful to receive Sara's passion and knowledge for yoga. I've learned so much from her over the years as I go into other classes remembering it was Sara that has taught me almost everything I know. Thank you Sara."
—Amy Vida, National Sales Director/Niche Media, Beverly Hills CA

"I love taking Sara's classes for the rigorous sequences that challenge my body and focus my mind. Her attention to breath and movement have helped me to evolve into a more calm and patient person outside of the yoga studio. I especially thank her for exposing me to the many wonderful spiritual arms of yoga, the rituals, the moon practices, etc. I never thought I would pay attention to full moons and Hindu Holidays. Ha!"
—Lauren Berman, Teacher, Santa Monica, CA

"Sara's yoga classes focus on learning the yoga and not so much the poses. She has an incredible knowledge that she instills into her class. Sitting down after savasana she asks us to close our eyes and she urges us to expand into the corners of the room and then into the street and then to realize or beware of the fact we are everywhere. Once you realize this, you will be happier!"
—David Young Wolff, Photographer, Santa Monica, CA

"I love Sara's class . . . so tough . . . there are two things I love about it . . . her voice, number one . . . it's so resonant and lovely . . . she puts you in these positions, sweat dripping, straining, you don't think you can stand it another second, then she talks, and something about her voice eases everything, it relaxes you into it, and you discover that you can go further and deeper . . . great gift . . . and I dig her singing at the end too.

"The second thing I like about her class is that she asks us to close our eyes . . . she's the only teacher I know who asks the class to really feel their way through the asanas. It's amazing what a simple thing like closing your eyes does. It builds a sense of honesty I think. I guess, as an actor, being aware of how it actually feels to do yoga is important, and Sara is so helpful and insightful about that."
—Tate Donovan, Actor, *Damages*

I've often thought about regaling Sara with praise and pranams. However, thought better of it. I wouldn't want to upset the delicate balance we have going: boss to employee, teacher to student, all-knowing big sister to begrudgingly grateful little sister, the Cheshire Cat to Alice in Wonderland. If Alice hadn't been so friggin' precocious, she may not have learned all those hard lessons. She thought she knew everything though, so down the rabbit hole she goes . . .

But that Sara would just not give up.

She can be so annoying sometimes.

"Ame, did you go to class today? "

"No."

"Are you going to?"

"No."

"Ame, do your practice."

"Ugh. I know. Hey Sar?"

"Yeah?"

"Thanks. I needed that. I'll see you in class."

Sara grew up in Mill Valley, California. That's in Marin County, just eight miles north of the Golden Gate Bridge. Marin is home to many of our favorite touchy feely people: Senator Barbara Boxer; Author Allan Watts; Fillmore West founder, Bill Graham; and my personal favorite, The Grateful Dead.

I grew up in suburban New Jersey, just six miles west of The George Washington Bridge. I spent most of my formative years going under-over, upper-back across that bridge, to and from the city, and the outer borough of Brooklyn where my grandparents are from.

In New York, the term "F–you" is a lot like "Aloha." It means "Hi," "Bye," "Thank You," "Good To See You," "By the way, your boyfriend sweats me," "Who, my boyfriend?" "Yeah, your boyfriend," and then of course, it also means "F–you."

In Mill Valley, you're probably ticketed and ordered to do community service, hugging the Redwood Trees in the Muir Woods, for using such foul language.

Sara's parents are good Brooklyn Jews from the block. I love hugging trees listening to The Dead. So there ya have it.

My dad is a white, Republican, middleclass, conservative, Vietnam era Navy veteran who spent thirty-two years commuting into the city to provide for his wife and daughter. Thirteen of those years were also spent serving on the River Edge Fire Department. He rescued cats from trees, helped old ladies cross the street, ran into approximately 1,100 burning buildings, pulled twenty or so burned bodies out of cars (including some of my classmates), engaged in about ten Hail Mary! "Surround and drowns" fireman moves and then sat atop Engine #2 each Christmas dressed as Santa, handing candy canes out to neighborhood kids. In his world, there's only so much room for the touchy feely stuff, and it showed up once a year riding a reindeer (or a fire truck, as the case may be).

This "toughen up" training has served me very well. I'm one of those annoying "I can do anything" people. A trait that has helped me persevere while putting together Ikea furniture, my nephew's toy fire truck and even an A List movie director's computer when a teamster accidentally ran over it with the wardrobe trailer.

This characteristic has NOT served me so well in all of my human relationships. It's difficult for me to admit to wrongdoings (because there aren't any), and God forbid I let anyone in. (Why would I want to? People are so annoying.)

Knock, knock, it's me, Sara.

Ugh. Not her again. Duck!

When I was 18, I hiked "The Long Trail," the 163.18 miles of the Appalachian Trail that runs through Vermont. My girlfriends and I carried 40 pounds in our backpacks. I also carried the freshmen 15. Less than halfway through our intended path, my swift, trim, hare-like trail mates burned out and quit. I turned into the tortoise. Slowly, but steadily, I won the race.

As a starving artist in New York City, I moved myself from 156th and Broadway to E. 23rd St. and 2nd Ave. on the subway. That's two transfers including the Times Square Station. I went in with a mid-August tan and little knowledge of the underground rails. I emerged early September pale as a ghost with a clear understanding of the city beneath the city. Thank God for monthly metro cards and the kindness of door-holding strangers.

Most impressively, I finished a stick of lip-gloss while following the band Phish across country in college. Anyone who has traveled in this manner can appreciate the organization, responsibility and dedication that requires.

When caught in the 2006 Blizzard that shut down New York City, producer Richard B. Lewis announced in front of an entire film crew, "If I ever had to be in the Donner Party, I would want you with me."

"So do you want me dead, or do you want to eat me, or both?"

"Neither! I want you to pull the cart. What is all that you are carrying?! Ask one of the guys to give you a hand."

"I'm good I can handle it, thanks."

You forgot your harmonium and your set is in five minutes? I'll be right back.

The wedding planner cancelled and you need someone to take over? I'm your girl.

The DP quit and the crew walked out? You need to replace them by tonight or blow your budget? Give me ten minutes.

The babysitter didn't show? What time is your gig? I'll be there at ten.

You haven't gotten laid in a year, and are climbing up the walls? Okay, I have a guy for you. Take these Toots and the Maytals tickets, call Brett and ask for extra anchovies.

Of course I'll proofread your screenplay, listen to your album, go to your comedy show . . .

What's that Lassie? Timmy fell in a well? I'll be right there.

Now, do these qualities make me an extremely efficient worker who has been blessed with amazing opportunities, experiences and meeting many dynamic people in the process?

Yes.

Does it make me an openhearted, kind and genuine person? Well . . .

Knock, knock, it's Sara.

Whaaaaaaaaat?!?!?!?!???

As I was saying, it doesn't leave a lot of time and space for all the touchy feely stuff. And then *boom,* a legitimate tragedy strikes and after I've flown in, called the funeral parlor, called the caterer, called the car service and the florist, filed the 501C3 so we can collect "in memory of" scholarship funds, gotten through the day, been sure all the immediates are well hydrated and home in bed with plates to heat up if they get hungry, I'm leveled.

Sound familiar, Wonder Women? I'm a product of my parents, their parents and the parents before them. Where I grew up you keep calm and carry on. New Yorkers are survivors. We don't sit around talking about our feelings. We pull ourselves up by the bootstraps, make posters that say "I Love New York Now More Than Ever" and go to work the next day. We're not going to let them win this. *We are stronger than THEY think.*

Then I get a call about an emergency quadruple by-pass, a cheating spouse or a lethal overdose and all bets are off. Where I'm from we're not taught how to talk about our feelings, take care of our minds, bodies, hearts and souls. Why would we? There's work to be done, cancer to cure, world peace to achieve and all that oil still polluting the gulf. I didn't know taking care of yourself was something people did until . . .

Knock, knock, its Sara.

Okay, you can come in now.

Ame?

Yeah?

Are you in here?

Uh huh.

I'm sorry about your friend.

It's okay.

You okay?

Yeah, I'm fine.

You don't look fine.

I'm fine.

Have you eaten?

No.

Do you need something to eat?

No, I'm okay thanks.

Here I brought you some green soup.

Oh, okay, thanks. Slurp, slurp.

Have you been to yoga?

Not since I got back.

Come to class tonight as my guest.

Okay, thanks.

And Ame?

Yeah?

It's all right to cry . . .

That Sara would just not give up.
She can be so annoying sometimes.
Thank God.

"Jesus Wept"

—JOHN 11:35

CHAPTER 7

The Practice

*"Healing does not mean going back to the way things were before,
but rather allowing what is now to move us closer to God."*

—Ram Dass

Stan Deland—Former Marine, Owner of Siddatech, Malibu, CA

Stan: There are different classifications of casualties, and there is a thing called golden hour. If you get someone medical treatment within one hour, their chances of survival go way up. There's "urgent," "routine," and "priority." Routine is a scratch or if someone is dead. It means there's not much you can do. Priority is kinda minor—they can walk by themselves, but need attention. Urgent is if someone has been shot five times and he's bleeding out or something like that. You can save him, but he's not going to live if he doesn't get medical attention. Sometimes there would be more than one guy at a time. I think as a battalion, we had 22 that died and 500 purple hearts.

There were guys that were pretty messed up, and the thing about it now is that those guys . . . okay, so you fix the physical injury, but . . . There was one guy, he was a corporal, he was getting out, he was going to go to college, he was gonna hike the Appalachian trail, he was going to do all these different things—he was going on to the rest of his life. He basically had one month left. I evac'ed him. He had been shot in the leg, he had been shot in the arm, a couple guys he was with, one of them had died at that point, and another guy we thought was going to be fine ended up dying of a blood clot. But this guy . . . that really got to me. I had liked the guy, I knew what he wanted to do, he was a smart kid . . . the mental emotional scars, it's much more subtle and it's not addressed as easily as the physical stuff.

Amy: I read that the psychological scars are really adding up. This year there have been 167 active duty suicides and the number is projected to be 200 by years' end. The rate doubled from June to July. Doubled!

Stan: Yeah, with a deployable unit they're like $18^1/_2$ years old at that point and they are going over there for seven months, coming back, going over again and guys are doing four or five deployments in a row. So all your nervous system knows after a while is high alert. It's just freak-out mode.

Amy: Is that why you started a yoga and meditation practice? I thought when you were at war you were supposed to be blowing shit up, day-dreaming about your best gal and cherry pie, not attaining Samadhi.

Stan: Well, that too. I remember being in Fallujah and I had just done this casualty evacuation. I was talking to our OPSO [Operations Officer] who really knew what the fuck he was doing and I had a lot of respect for him, and he was asking what was going on. I was out in the field and was sort of the go-between these guys. I felt like I was doing a great job and I was able to do my thing and be effective in this pretty intense scenario, but then he was asking me questions and I was sweating. That had been going on with me for a while—I would start to get anxious and it would snowball into this situation where I could not be present what-soever. So I was like, what the fuck? Why does that happen to me?

When I got back it was January 2005. I was dating this woman who took me to this alternative healing place. So I thought okay, I'll clean up my diet, I'll see a chiropractor, get some acupuncture, yadda yadda. So I did that stuff and felt a little better all around. That girl broke up with me. I was bummed about that, and one of the guys I was lieutenant with on that first peacetime deployment had hung himself, and I [was the one who] found him. I went to Iraq once, then that happened, I went to Iraq again, and I had never really dealt with that at all. So those are three very obvious things to me. I was like, I want to change this in my life. Or, I want to deal with the trauma. And it wasn't even really the trauma of being in Iraq—it was those other things that were bigger deals to me personally.

Amy: Those are all compounded symptoms of emotional trauma though, right? You hold it all together for so long and then the levee breaks?

Stan: Yeah, it's a pretty basic thing. One's nervous system gets to a point where it is just overwhelmed with too much of whatever kind of stress and it basically just keeps freaking out and I don't think that is just something that fixes itself over time. I don't believe that time necessarily heals things. More things get layered on top. But that doesn't mean that it is gone from the person's experience and the nervous system is what connects the deeper sense of being with the physical experience.

It's just a question of, is a person even able to get to the point where they can make good decisions and do things that can help themselves? If they are too hemmed up, they can't. They are basically underwater in general, then it's just a tough situation. I mean, obviously, with the suicide rate there are guys that, ya know, are really underwater. They cannot—they do not know how to cope with the experience. There is some sort of dissonance or disconnect going on.

Amy: What are some of the ways you have connected yourself to prevent getting to that point?

Stan: I went to Geoffrey [healer and now his business partner]. He said, "We're going to clear all the bullshit, we're going to restore personal power and you're going to figure out how stuff works." Loving the marine efficiency of that mentality I was like, sign me up dude, I'm there. It was yoga, meditation, acupuncture, energy work, different modalities and Bach Flower Essences, which as you know is what I do now. I felt a lot of positive change in myself. This whole other world opened up for me. As most people are when they are just learning something, you want to tell everyone about it. You want to get them to do it.

Amy: (Self-conscious laugh) Oh, you mean like telling everyone how great yoga is for a broken heart?

Stan: (Laughs) Yeah, like that! Anyone who doesn't buy into it, thinks this stuff is hocus pocus, I recommend they take Vinnie Marino's Yoga Class [in LA] seven days a week. I did *Natrum Muriaticum* in an insane regimen that wouldn't be allowed by most homeopaths. It was the first thing I did—but that was the Marine in me. Some people don't need to make it hard on themselves.

Amy: I get it. Hard, fast, most challenging—best result.

Stan: Yeah, but even more than that. It's something to let go of your attachment to at some point. Let go of suffering.

Amy: Oorah Siddhartha.

Stan: Oorah Heartbreak Yoga.

Amy: Thanks for your service, Stan.

   We hug.

Ashley Turner, Yoga Teacher and Psychologist specializing in Neurobiology, Jungian Psychology, Ayurveda, Tantra, Shamanism and Priestess work, Santa Monica, CA

One of the most important tools for us as modern day yogis is to learn how to stay in our body and stay connected to what we're feeling instead of disassociating, so yoga gives us really practical tools. It's thematic psychology to breathe with it. To stay with intensity, whether it's contraction muscularly; holding patterns (some that may be habitual); residual defense mechanisms that the body is carrying from trauma or stress; or anxiety, but also learning how to go in and very specifically, learning how to unwind those patterns using the breath, to stay with the feeling. Maybe it's an emotional feeling that is coming up, agitation, irritation, this general discomfort that we experience when we are going through anything that we don't like, that we don't find (quote, unquote) pleasurable. So, yoga gives us the very clear tools to learn how to stay anchored and grounded in our bodies, which is the key to healing. You can't heal what you can't feel.

So instead of disassociating, turning toward any sort of addictive behavior (whether it's the big five: alcohol, drugs, sex, work, money, or something more subtle, such as our addiction to fear, our addiction to self-doubt, insecurity), it is really creating some space in our bodies, but also learning how to create space in our minds, between the thought-forms, so we can more objectively observe—what are our habits? what are our tendencies? And then choose to stay with and learn how to tolerate the intensity of suffering. And we all suffer! Whether it's grieving, sadness, disappointment, heartache, insecurity, or all of those. How do we learn to tolerate that experience, work with it, get curious about it, instead of pushing it away, fearing it, cutting it off?

It's very intense work. It's not easy and it's definitely the road less traveled.

Tommy Rosen—Co-creator of the Tadasana Yoga & Music Festival, Yoga for Recovery Teacher, Venice, CA

When you get sober, your chosen medicine is taken away. You are left with all of your core issues and it is likely you will try to find other ways to avoid yourself. What you want is to find connection, ease, peace of mind and calmness, but you have no idea how to get these. Yoga nudges you along a path to all those things and it also helps to process stuck energy out of the body. Yoga helps you to get the issues out of your tissues and this should be of interest to any human being whether they struggle with acute addiction or not.

My addictions were like a force field surrounding my un-healed self. I needed to heal the trauma that resulted in disconnection, dis-ease and an internal sense of lack so powerful that it caused me to self-medicate again and again even in spite of disastrous consequences. Indeed, since addiction does all that it can to dismantle a person's life, one must take a holistic approach to putting that life back together. Yoga has been a key ingredient on my path to recovery from addiction. I call it the addiction buster. If you practice with a gifted teacher, you will catch the consciousness of transformation and it will become possible to heal in ways you might not have imagined possible.

Whereas today yoga serves me as a path from dis-ease into ease, it just as effectively serves a person who is looking for a kick-ass workout or someone else who wants to heal from an injury or someone else who wants to work on stress management and calming the mind. It meets the practitioner where they are at, gives them what they need and nudges them toward their next step of "becoming" along their unique destiny path. I've turned to the practice of yoga to give me each of these things at various points along my journey. Yoga has never let me down. Now, as a teacher of people in recovery from addiction, I apply yoga to the situation because it continues to deliver on its promise to lift us out of the darkness of addiction and into the light of infinity.

And that's pretty badass, if you ask me!

Dana Flynn—Co-creator, Laughing Lotus Yoga Center

There's this old interview with Al Green when someone asked him, "How do you come up with your songs?"

He said "Well, when I wrote 'Let's Stay Together,' or 'Here I Am,' " one of his great songs, "it came out of the clear blue sky."

The clear blue sky means you show up and you practice every day. Even when you don't want to. Even when you are in pain. Especially when you are in pain. When you look at a Picasso Painting, you sense that Picasso's work has changed and you are grateful for that. You wouldn't want him to forever be the same. We wouldn't have seen the blue period!

You know, the Matisse cutouts that the artist Henri Matisse is most famous for were done when he was bedridden and could barely see—at the very end of his life, and yet they are some of his most memorable!

Like, we don't know when we keep showing up what our canvas is going to look like tomorrow, or next week, but we have to keep showing up.

Arthur Klein—Emmy winning director of documentary, *Y Yoga Movie*

It was early September 2001 and I was traveling around the country directing a TV special honoring great public school teachers when 9/11 happened.

A week earlier, I had picked up a schedule for Power Yoga, a donation-based yoga studio in Santa Monica around the corner from my office. So as I sat there still in a state of shock, I looked down, saw the schedule, and left my office in the middle of the day to head to a 1:30 p.m. yoga class.

I grew up in Manhattan watching the towers being built. When the towers collapsed, so did my understanding of the world. Who knew what was going to happen next? I just wanted to find some peace, so that's where I went.

Dana Pustetta—Director of Photography, *Animal Planet*

The boardwalk in seaside was one of my parents' first dates in 1961. The childhood memories from there were endless. I remember a double date my senior year of high school, riding that roller coaster. I was now looking at it half-submerged in the Atlantic Ocean. The boardwalk where I had celebrated my 20th and 30th birthdays was decimated. Every decade of my life held memories from a place that was wiped away overnight.

I promised Nicole I would take her there someday. She had called me two nights before she passed, and I rushed off the phone. I rarely regret things I do; I find it's the things I don't do that I end up regretting. I never told her how much I really loved her, how she meant the world to me, and it still breaks my heart.

Now they're both gone.

Can I take you up on that offer to teach me yoga? I can't put it off any longer.

> *"When the student is ready, the teacher will appear."*
> —BUDDHIST PROVERB

> *(When the teacher is ready, the student will appear.)*

> *The Light Within Me*
> *Sees the Light Within You.*

> *Xo*

Fifty million Elvis fans can't be wrong, and there's got to be something to a practice that has sustained relevance over the course of 5,000 years.

We call yoga a practice out of reverence and respect for these ancient teachings, their lineage, and the teachers on the path before us. We don't ever "perfect" yoga. Even the Indian Sadhus born into families of yogis, twisted up into a pretzel, have not perfected yoga. We are all simply practicing yoga.

Sara Ivanhoe is my maha (main) yoga asana teacher. Her maha yoga asana teacher is Erich Schiffmann. That makes him my grand teacher. Something like your Big Big in a sorority.

Out of respect for my teacher, her teachers, their teachers all the way back to the original practitioners of India in 1500 BCE, I personally begin my practice with a prayer of respect and gratitude to those human beings, the intuitive teachers within them, and the intuitive teacher within me. That small voice that says, "*Psst . . . get on your yoga mat.*

You'll feel better if you do." That prayer is called the Guru Stotram and it goes like this:

Guru Brahma

Guru Vishnu

Guru Devo Maheshwara

Guru Sak Sha

Param Brahma

Tasmayi Shri Guruvay Namah

Tasmayi Shri Guruvay Namah

To negate any televangelist voodoo images your mind might be presenting you with, the word "guru" does not mean "call in now, give me all your money, the deed to your home, your first born and your soul." It actually just means "dispeller of darkness." Your guru is whoever or whatever dispels the darkness from your heart and soul.

We all have some darkness, hurt or disappointment. What belief, dogma or physical representation helps to shine-a-light and alleviate it? No propaganda here. Much like a midnight buffet in Vegas, I'm just laying it all out. Your plate may be piled with oysters, while the bride-to-be goes head first into the Bananas Foster. Only you know what, and how much is right for you.

The forthcoming terms of yoga asana postures are in Sanskrit. Sanskrit is the ancient Indo-Aryan Language of India. Vedic Sanskrit dates back to the Rig Veda sometime around 1500 BCE. It is from this corpus, many of our modern day yoga terms, allegories, hymns and prayers are derived.

The physical practice the populous of the U.S. refers to as "Yoga" is actually called "Asana." It is one of but eight limbs, or eight "Steps" of yoga as defined by Patanjali in "The Yoga Sutras of Patanjali," the first recorded manual of yoga written in 200 BCE.

The first two limbs are called the "Yamas" and "Niyamas." They are a code of moral and mental conduct for the aspirant's behavior. In their most rudimentary form they are as follows:

The First Limb:
The Yamas—Attitudes Toward Others

Ahimsa: non-violence, kindness toward all beings

Satya: truth

Asteya: to take nothing that doesn't belong to us

Brahmacharya: sexual responsibility

Aparigraha: taking only what is necessary

The Second Limb:
The Niyamas—Attitude Toward Oneself

Sauca: Cleanliness, inner (the mind, proper function of the body and its organs)

Samtosa: Modesty and being content with what we have.

Tapas: Keeping fit with particular attention to the physical body

Svadhya: Self-examination

Isvarapranidhana: Directly translated means "To lay all your actions at the feet of God." Meaning, do your best, adhere to the Yamas and Niyamas and know that the rest (the outcome) is up to a higher power.

The Third Limb:
Yoga Asana—The Practice of Physical Postures

Patanjali describes yoga as "Yogash citta vritti ni ro dah."

"Yoga is the ability to direct the mind exclusively toward an object and sustain that direction without any distractions."

Living master teacher who has been practicing for more than 78 years, B.K.S. Iyengar, who was taught by the legendary Sri Tirumalai Krishnamacharya in Mysore, India, in the 1930s reflects:

"Yoga, an ancient but perfect science, deals with the evolution of humanity. This evolution includes all aspects of one's being, from bodily health to self-realization. Yoga means union—the union of body with consciousness and consciousness with the soul."

The Word "Yoga" literally translates as "to yoke" or "to yuje," "to join." In the physical practice of yoga asana we are yoke-ing, yuje-ing and joining breath with movement, the higher self with the human self, the pleasure with the pain, the male with the female, a little bit country with a little bit rock n' roll. It is a practice of melting the hard edges and looking within to find the greater consciousness that may have been buried beneath.

In *Heartbreak Yoga,* we are yoke-ing heartbreak, with the innate knowledge that is already inside of you—the part of your heart that knows what to let go of, what to be with, what to grieve, what to be relieved by, what to release and what to love more.

Living saint and humanitarian Sri Sri Mātā Amāritānandamayī Devī leads by example, teaching:

"There is always a divine message hidden in the seemingly negative experiences we go through. We just have to penetrate beneath the surface of a situation and the message will be revealed."

May you find the strength to penetrate beneath the surface of this experience. *You are stronger than you think.*

One of the strongest women I know is Yogalosophy's Mandy Ingber. I asked what she thought of this concept of "Heartbreak Yoga"—joining together what hurts with what is beautiful beneath it. She contemplated and responded with the following:

"Even as he was dying, my father was completely inspiring. He would say, 'Other than this cancer, this is the healthiest I've ever been.' He would also say that the yoga helped to alleviate the symptoms of the cancer and the chemotherapy. One of the greatest gifts he said he received in his last days was the gift of receiving. How open his heart had become to others during this vulnerable time. What a gift, to show up as we are. Today is a new day. This is the day that I have. Exactly as I am. Right now. Today I show up, brokenhearted . . . and full of life. How many mornings have I woken up and taken this day for granted when life was just too much? I often feel too vulnerable with my heartbreaks (and I have many). But how to open up and offer my vulnerability to the Universe and give thanks for another day, that is the lesson yoga offers."

So, we have THIS day. What are we going to do with it? Use it to open, and ripen and dive deeper into ourselves, into our heartbreak and our healing? Or avoid it and push it off another day? I'll be on the mat. Hope to see you there.

Common Excuses and Misconceptions for Not Practicing Yoga

"I'm not flexible."
And I can't rip a Les Paul like Slash. You know why? Because I don't practice guitar scales every day. Sara Ivanhoe reminds us, "Whatever we practice, we get good at." Are we practicing finding flexibility or are we practicing making excuses? The Sistine Chapel ceiling took four years to paint, but it is one of Michelangelo's finest offerings and his legacy. Things take time, patience, and a cultivated sense of participation. Don't worry, it won't take four years to feel the benefits of yoga asana. *You are what you seek. You are stronger than you think.*

"I'm out of shape. I won't be able to do any of it."
Yoga is meant to make you feel good, not bad. Every practice (if taught properly) begins with a warm up and a cool down. There are resting poses for you to retreat into if you have reached your limit, or if you just plain don't feel like doing something. No, you don't have to balance on your head in full lotus during your first class. In fact, a responsible teacher wouldn't let you.

"I'm too old."

Amy: Whatever. Julia Child was thirty-four when she first learned to cook.

Cheyanne: I didn't do my first handstand until I was fifty-one.

Amy: How old were you when you began your yoga asana practice?

Cheyanne: Forty-eight.

Amy: Exactly my point.

"Isn't yoga a religion?"

No, yoga is not a religion. It has roots in Hinduism, however practitioners of all faiths come together to practice the art of connecting to their own bodies. Kim Dumas teaches a wonderful Christian "Three in One Yoga" in the Bible Belt. She wanted to make the benefits of yoga accessible to those who were misinformed and fearful of its intention and benefits. With her perfect southern drawl (and finely sculpted bod) Kim begins class with the following Bible verse:

"A heart at peace gives life to the body."
—PROVERBS 14:30

"I shave my armpits and don't wear Patchouli Oil."

Los Angeles is the entertainment capital of the world and hosts 300 yoga classes daily. Students in those classes are network executives, studio moguls and your household names: actors, actresses, rock stars, musicians, models, former models, wannabe models. They are the writers of your TV shows, famed super-agents, Oscar-winning producers, composers, documentarians, teachers, moms, nannies, students, artists, doctors, lawyers and even cowboys. This cross section engages in yoga to manage the physical and mental demands of their lifestyle. Many pull up to class in their Jaguars before dinner at The Ivy. I can assure you, the only one among them who smells like Patchouli is Russell Brand. (And he wears it well, so who cares?)

"I don't want to 'OM.' It's weird."
You don't have to. Please take from the following what works for you and leave the rest behind (a recurring theme).

My Understanding of Om and Everything After

Have you ever been in an elevator alone and picked your nose, fixed a wedgie, or changed your clothes? What does it feel like? Have you ever entered an elevator and been totally creeped out by the copy guy cooing at you from the corner? What does it feel like? How about when you hop in that same elevator and find the hot guy from human resources pushing all your buttons? What does it feel like?

Would you now agree that people, places and things can contain different vibes? "Aum" is the sacred symphonic syllable resonating with all of it—perceived good/bad, up/down, in/out, penthouse/basement, Yankees/Red Socks, it's all just two sides of the same cosmic coin.

In early Vedantic literature, we learn that "Aum" is the vibration of the supreme divine all-encompassing consciousness first taking form as sound.

"A" resonates with Brahman Shakti, Creation; "U" resonates with Vishnu Shakti, Preservation; "M" resonates with Shiva Shakti, Destruction and Liberation. This birth-life-death cycle is present in all aspects of life on Earth.

Therefore, when we chant "Aum" or "Om" as it is now commonly called, we are not necessarily phoning home to E.T., hoping the Mother Ship beams us up—we are aligning with the vibration of the universe and the energy that creates, maintains and destroys it. Additionally, like a first chair violinist about to attempt the Elgar, we are tuning up to the conditions of that concert stage, classroom, or energetic current.

Do you want to try one just for fun? C'mon, I won't tell.

1. Let out ALL of the air in your lungs—empty out completely.

2. Now take a big deep breath in, down to your lower lungs. Relax into fullness.

Please note: Dramatically inhaling your shoulders up to your ears and puffing out your cheeks is not taking a deep breath into your lower lungs, it's just dramatically inhaling your shoulders up to your ears and puffing out your cheeks. Ya feel me? Remember what your elementary school teachers used to tell you? "When you cheat, you only cheat yourself." Want to try again?

Take a big deep breath down to your lower lungs. Relax into fullness.

3. On the exhale say, sing, chant or chime out the sacred syllable "Aum" until all of the air has expelled from your lungs.

Yes, it's that easy.
There's no place like Om.

Common Questions

"What should I wear?"

Anything you are comfortable in. Know that in many of the postures we are folding forward and/or positioned in a way that most loose T-shirts will hang over your head. I recommend wearing something snug and/or wearing two layers, tucking one of them in. For you dudes, double shorts. Please, just trust me. Double shorts. Of course in some parts of India, Nepal, and West Hollywood the practice is done naked. And then there's the famous "Kama Sutra" but one step at a time. Let's get you on the mat first.

"What do I need?"

Yoga Mat: If you are doing a home practice, a flat clean surface is great. If you have a non-skid yoga mat even better. My favorite mats are made by Gaiam or Manduka. Please be sure to have bare feet to avoid the slipping and sliding socks can cause.

Water Bottle: It is always nice to have a water bottle. Serious practitioners limit liquid intake during the practice, to keep their inner fire their "Agni" ignited, but do what feels right for you!

Towel: You may work up a good sweat and enjoy having a towel. It is also helpful in restorative poses when you need a little help to get into the sweet relaxation spot.

Props: If you decide to invest in your yoga practice (your physical, mental and spiritual health) a yoga block is a great prop. It helps you move into positions that may not be accessible to you otherwise—*yet*. A strap, bolster and blanket may enhance your experience as well. But I would start with the block. The body is where it is. You will know what is right for you.

Open Mind: Take it easy on yourself . . . don't forget the first Yama is Ahimsa, non-violence and kindness. That's means even to yourself. Crazy, right? No beating yourself up! That's a rule!

"And you? When will you begin that
long journey into yourself?"

—RUMI

हेअर्त्ब्रेअक्योग

CHAPTER 8

Yoga Poses

THIS PRACTICE WAS CREATED WITH THE DHĀRAŅĀ (FOCUS) of yoke-ing a standard complete yoga asana practice, with mindful awareness of healing the heart. Please note: Poses will repeat as they do in all vinyasa flow sequences.

SETTING A SANKALPA

A sankalpa is an intention, a wish or a resolve. It is a positive, affirmative phrase "I am at peace," "I am healing," "I am letting go of heartache," "I feel whole." The sixth limb of Patanjali's yoga sutras is "Dharana" focus. What is your heart longing for? What is it best for you to focus on? From deep within your heart find your resolve. Once you have that wish, that intention, the person, place, thing, feeling, idea, intention you would like to dedicate your practice to, reduce it down to a word, picture or phrase you can call upon. Then "Set" the intention. With your palms at your heart. Seal this secret inside.

1. Come into a comfortable cross-legged seated position (Sukhasana/ Easy Pose) or (Padmasana/Lotus pictured at left)

2. Bring your palms together in "prayer position" at your heart. This is called Anjali mudra. Anjali means "offering." Mudra means "seal." Therefore, when we bring our palms together at our hearts, and get clear with our mind, we are literally sealing that thought, that intention into our heart.

UJJAYI BREATH

One of the key aspects of a yoga practice is connecting breath with movement. If this is your first yoga practice, just allow the breath to guide you. Perhaps this is the first time you have placed your attention on the breath. That's okay! Remember, yoga is meant to nourish and calm. There is no "right way"/"wrong way."

Ultimately we want to be using what the yogis call an Ujjayi breath. The ujjayi breath sounds like the waves of the ocean or Darth Vader. Ujjayi breath is translated as the "Victorious" as it is most energizing and calming. This long and smooth (Dirga & suksma) sounding breath is created by gently constricting the glottis (the back of the throat). The slight tension creates an ocean sound as you inhale and exhale.

Try to do five Ujjayi breaths now.

If you were successful and can feel this "Victorious" powerful breath, fantastic. If not, you will get it when you are supposed to. Taking five deep, calm, nourishing breaths is more than most people do to care for themselves all day. Congratulations, Yogi. You are on your way!

Balasana (Child's Pose)

1. Kneel on the floor, allowing your big toes to touch.

2. Sit back on to your heels.

3. Allow your knees to separate hips distance.

4. Take in a nice inhale.

5. On the exhale begin to lay your torso between your thighs, moving toward the ground as far as is comfortable to you. (Feel free to place a folded blanket, or towel beneath you for additional support, as Jo has done here.)

6. Lay your hands out in front of you, or along your sides with palms face up.

7. Allow the forehead to relax toward the ground. You may want to rest your head on a pillow made from your hands, a towel or a blanket. For more challenge, lower your forehead on to the ground.

8. Invite your shoulders to let go into the ground.

9. Feel your sit bones reaching back, and finding length between your forehead and your sit bones.

10. Stay here a minimum of three to ten breaths.

11. Extend both arms in front of you with your hands shoulder distance, fingers pointing straight ahead. Take one last breath here before moving into the next pose.

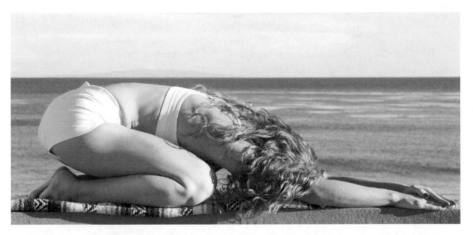

Child's pose is always here for you!

Balasana is a resting pose. It is meant to help you recover a sense of safety. Sometimes when we're raw, beat up, hurt, bent and barely want to get out from under the covers, just breathing in child's pose can feel like a triathlon. That's okay. Balasana is here for you. Retreat into this wonderful nourishing pose. This is one of only two postures the body can fully rest in without using any muscles. Enjoy it! You may want to picture any unneeded thoughts draining out of your third eye center (the ajna chakra), between the eyes. You may want to feel the Earth holding you safely in the palm of her hand. You may just want to crawl into Child's Pose and cry your eyes out. That's great! That what it is here for. Child's Pose is our friend. Play "getting to know you" games with this wonderful pose. It is here when you need it.

Bitilasana/Marjaryasana (Cow/Cat Pose)

Cow

1. Come on to your hands and knees in a neutral tabletop position. Hands below the shoulders. Knees beneath the hips. Fingers are spread and pointing forward. Head relaxes. Gaze looks at the floor.

2. On an inhale, lift your chest and sitbones toward the ceiling. Relax your belly. Let anything you are holding in your abdomen just go. Let it hang out—no one is looking!

3. Lift your head, allow the neck to open.

4. Breathe deep into the low belly. Feel the collar bones spread. Allow an opening in the front of the body.

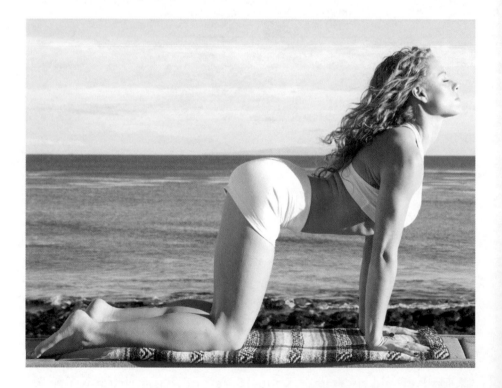

Cat

1. On the exhale, round your spine toward the ceiling.

2. Let go on your head and neck.

3. Breathe into the back, locate the back side of your heart cavity as it reaches up toward the sky.

4. Feel a great stretch in your upper back, allow any held tension to just break open and release.

   • On an Inhale move back into Cow

   • On the exhale move into cat

   • Continue this for 5–10 breaths

Cow/Cat poses massage the entire nervous system by activating the spine. It helps to unlock blocks of stagnant energy and stimulates the kidneys and adrenal glands (often activated by the worry over a heartbreak).

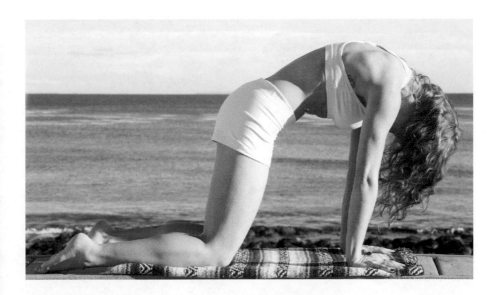

After you've done a few rounds of Cat/Cow come to rest in **Child's pose**.
   See! Child's pose is always here for you!
   Doesn't it feel good to listen to your body?

सूर्यनमस्कार

SŪRYA NAMASKĀRA (SALUTATIONS TO THE SUN)

Tadasana with Anjali Mudra Variation (Mountain Pose)

1. Bring your feet together at the front of your mat.

2. Bring your palms together at your heart.

3. Check back in with your sankalpa.

4. Feel your own strength. Feel the Earth supporting you.

Utthita Hasta in Tadasana

1. On an inhale, bring your arms up over your head.

2. Tip your head back slightly.

3. Feel your chest opening, allowing light to come in.

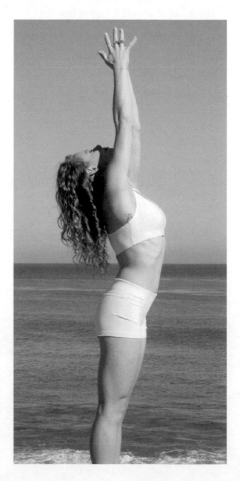

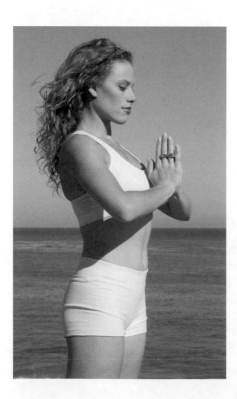

Uttanasana (Forward Fold)

1. With a flat back, slightly bend the knees, extend the arms out to the sides like an airplane. On an exhale, slowly fold your body down toward the Earth.

2. Place your hands at either side of your feet—it's okay if they don't reach!

3. Keep a slight bend in the knees.

4. Let go in the head and the neck.

5. Open the mouth.

6. Allow the tongue to hang out.

7. Let go in the jaw.

8. Release any tensions in the neck and shoulders.

9. Feel your heart through your back.

Ardha-Uttanasana

1. Keep a slight bend in the knees, fingers touch the floor, or place your hands in the middle of your shins.

2. With the knees bent, so the spine can elongate, on an inhale, lead with the heart and rise to a flat back. Chest reaches forward. Shoulders pull back and away from the ears.

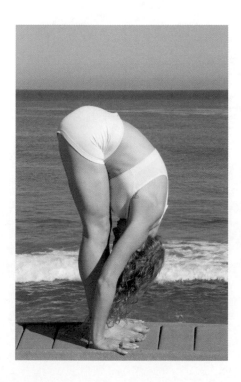

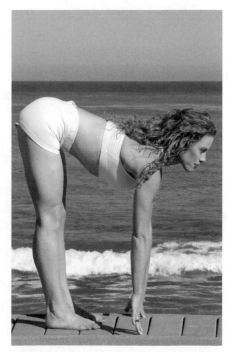

Kumbhakasana (Plank Pose)

1. On an exhale, bend your knees enough so your hands can reach the floor.

2. Step your feet toward the back of the mat.

3. Bring your body into a straight line, like a plank of wood.

This can be an extremely challenging pose. Feel free to release the knees on to the ground for support. You will be building upper body and abdominal strength—just like Xena, Wonder Woman and She-ra!

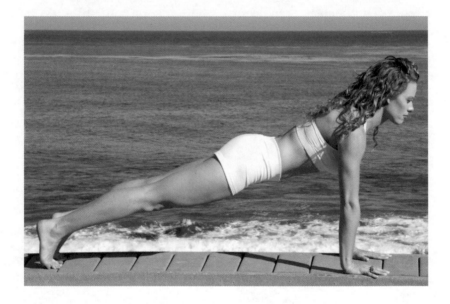

Chaturanga Dandasana

1. Continue to exhale while lowering yourself down to the Earth slowly, in a straight line. Chest lands first, belly should be the last thing to touch.

2. Elbows stay hugged into the body.

3. Hover a few inches above the ground—or lower all the way down!

4. Feel free to lower the knees to the ground for support.

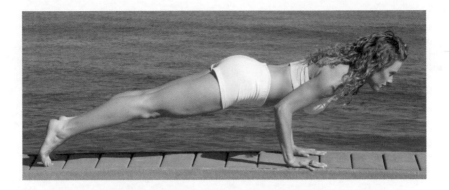

Urdhva Mukha Shvanasana or Salamba Bhujangasana (Updog or Sphinx)

Updog (top)

1. On an inhale, let your heart lead, up and open.

2. Tops of your feet press down, thighs lift, belly is in, draw the tailbone toward the floor. Leading with the heart, chest lifts.

3. Elbows are slightly bent, under shoulder and parallel.

4. Head tilts back slightly, opening throat and chest, shoulders should draw together behind you.

5. Don't forget to breathe. :)

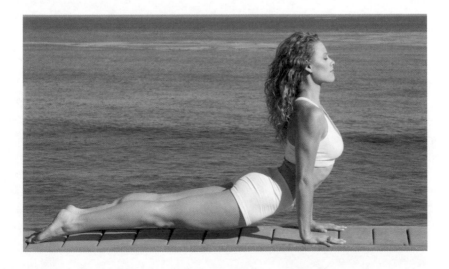

Sphinx (bottom)

1. On an inhale, let your heart lead, up and open.

2. Palms remain rooted into the floor under your shoulders.

3. Hug the elbows back, opening your shoulders .

4. Press the tops of the feet and thighs into the ground.

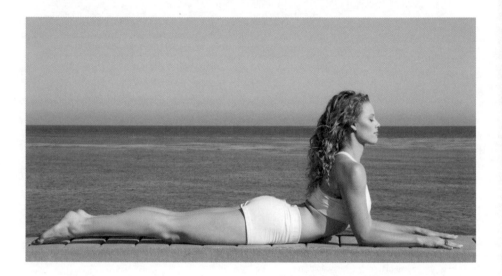

Updog and Sphinx are great for opening the heart. If you are rigid and achy and don't feel much like opening your heart, even a tiny little baby cobra move will help to alleviate some of the energetic tension you hold here. These poses help to alleviate stress and fatigue; however, backbends are NOT the place to push your body. Take it slow, be gentle on yourself and allow the heart to open in its own time. In every backbend do your best to aim the backbend, (the challenge and the work) into the upper back where the heart is.

Adho Mukha Shvanasana (Downward Facing Dog Pose)

1. Tuck the toes under and exhale, pushing back into downward facing dog pose.

2. Feet are hips distance and parallel.

3. Hands are shoulder distance, fingers point straight ahead and are spread wide. Press the inner edges of the palms, rooting into the Earth.

4. Begin with the knees bent and draw the hips, back and up away from the hands, elongating the spine. Feel free to stay here.

5. For more challenge try pressing the heels towards the floor. The legs moving toward straight. Most people find it challenging to have the legs and back straight so feel free to keep a bend in the knees.

6. Let go of your head and neck, give everything a shake, let go of any tension or holding in the shoulder, neck, jaw, tongue.

7. Let all the thoughts drain out of the crown of your head.

8. Hold it here for 3–15 full breaths—into the low belly!

9. Exhale fully. At the bottom of the exhale, inhale to move into the Ardha Uttanasana position (see page 117).

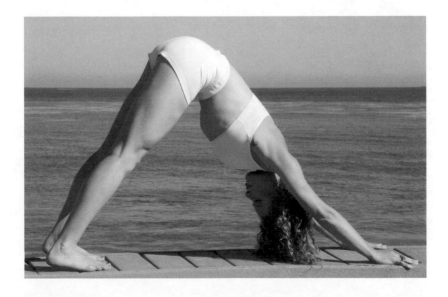

Ardha-Uttanasana

1. Heart lifts and chest lifts on an inhale

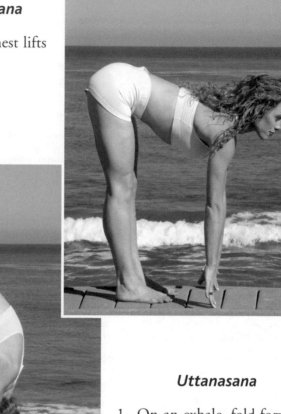

Uttanasana

1. On an exhale, fold forward.

2. Again, let go in the shoulders, neck, jaw, ears, mouth; let go of any thoughts or feelings that are not serving your highest good.

Utthita Hasta in Tadasana

1. On an inhale, reach the arms out to the sides and reach up with a flat back.

2. Arms reach up and over the head.

3. Head tips back slightly, heart and chest open.

4. Bring your palms together above your head.

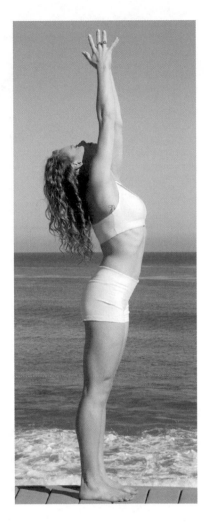

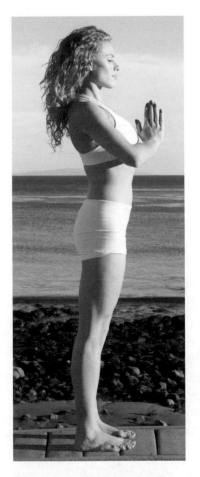

Tadasana with Anjali Mudra Variation

1. Bring your feet together at the front of your mat.

2. Bring your palms together at your heart.

3. Breathe into the heart center.

4. Remember your sankalpa, your resolve.

वरिभद्रसनईसे उएन्चे

VIRABHADRASANA II SEQUENCE (WARRIOR POSES)

Virabhadrasana II (Warrior II)

1. Stand at the top of your mat.

2. Step your right foot toward the back of the mat, in a heel arch alignment, allow the right foot to land about 4–5 feet behind at a 45–90 degree angle.

3. Take a nice big inhale in and on the exhale the front, left knee extends forward over the ankle.

4. Raise the arms until they are parallel to the ground. Shoulder blades reach down.

5. Stay here for 5–15 breaths.

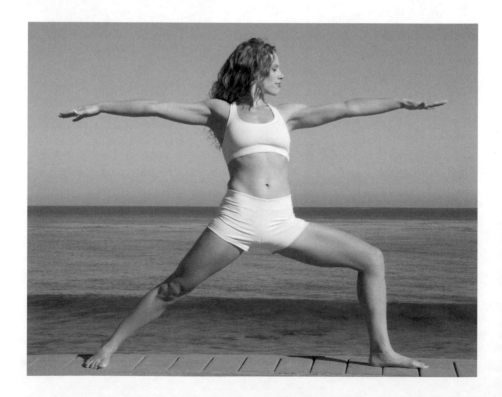

Reverse Virabhadrasana (Reverse Warrior Pose)

1. Right arm reaches down right back leg and rests either above or below the knee.

2. Left arm reaches up into the sky, allowing the chest to open

3. Be sure to maintain alignment. Left knee stacks on top of the left ankle.

4. Hold it for 5–15 breaths.

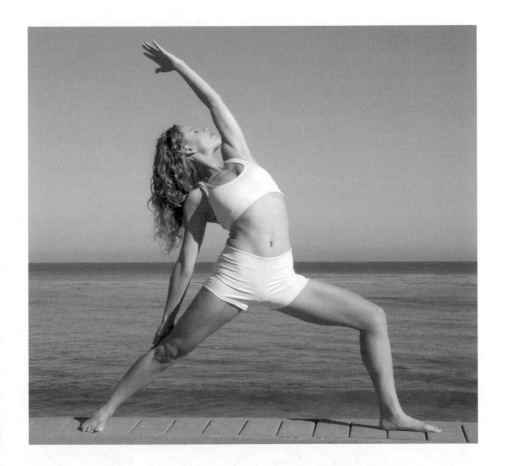

Utthita Parsvakonasana (Extended Side Angle Pose)

1. On the exhale, place your left arm down to thigh. For more challenge, your hands can come to rest on the floor either inside or outside of the front foot, rooting down into the ground.

2. Extend the right hand, up over the head, creating one long line on the right side of the body. Foot grounding into the earth, hand reaches up to the sun (be sure not to collapse your bottom shoulder).

3. Breathe into anywhere you might feel some tension, blocking, or holding.

Benefits include stretching and opening the chest muscles, shoulders and neck, building strength and balance.

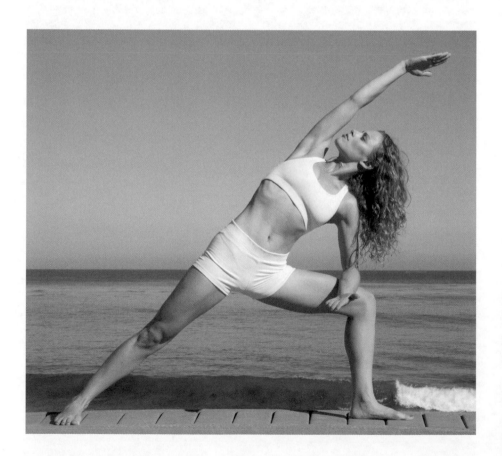

Virabhadrasana II Sequence Right Side (Warrior II Sequence)

Now repeat this entire sequence on side two:

- Virabhadrasana II

- Reverse Virabhadrasana

- Utthita Parsvakonasana

- Virabhadrasana II

Once you have learned it within your body, you may want to repeat the sequences anywhere from 3–5 times. The cardiovascular benefits are guaranteed to boost endorphins in your body, moving out some of the sadness or heartbreak. You will feel great!

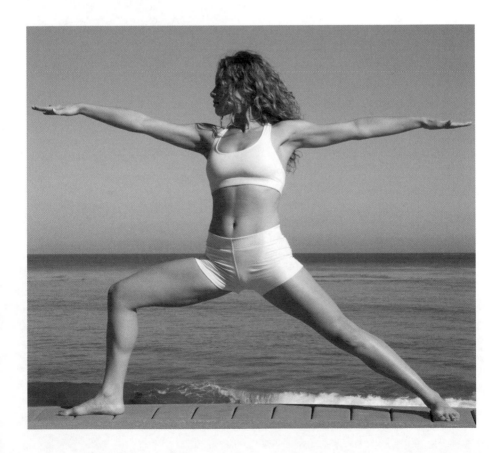

Utthita Trikonasana (Extended Triangle Pose)

1. Begin with both feet at the top of the mat. Palms together at the heart, in Tadasana Anjali Mudra Variation (see page 127). Step the right foot $3^1/_2$–4 feet behind in a heel to arch alignment.

2. Take an inhale.

3. On the exhale extend your torso over your left leg.

4. Hand reaches on to your leg, the floor or a block (shown here).

5. Right arm reaches up into the air.

6. Elongate the spine. Rotate chest towards the sky. Shoulder away from the ears. Be sure the chest is open. Heart always leads.

7. Breathe here for 5–15 breaths.

8. Exhale fully. On an inhale, lead with the chest and come to standing upright. Exhale, bring the back foot to the front of the mat. Land in Tadasana. Take a breath. Repeat on side 2.

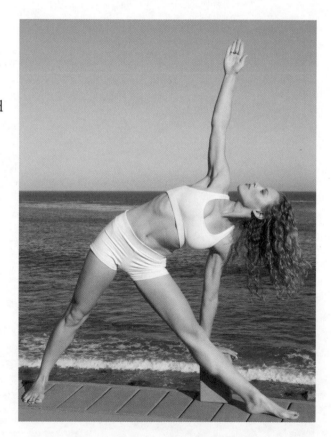

Prasarita Padottanasana (Wide-legged Forward Fold)

1. Bring your feet about $3^1/_2$ feet apart (wider is easier).

2. Be sure not to lock the knees.

3. Take an inhale, and on the exhale fold forward.

4. You may want to reach your arms down to the ground, or have each arm grab opposite elbows.

5. Let go of ALL the holding in the back of your head and neck. Allow your shoulders to release.

6. Perhaps shake your head and neck.

7. Again, allow any thoughts that are not serving you just to drain out of the crown of your head.

8. Maybe open your mouth, allowing your tongue to hang out.

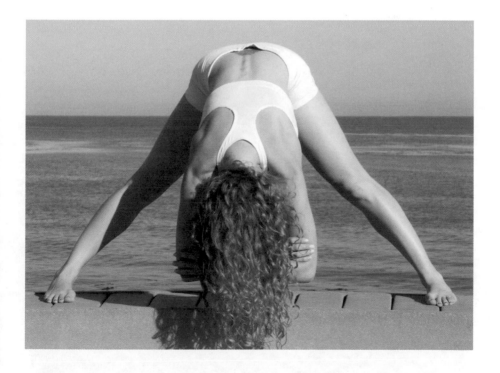

REAFFIRMING A SENSE OF SELF

Modified Navasana (Boat Pose)

No one really likes Boat Pose, but no one likes being unfit for bikini season either; so do it with me, folks . . .

1. Sit on your mat, with your legs out in front of you.

2. Now, bend your knees toward the ceiling, placing your feet flat on the floor.

3. Lift your heart, and chest, shoulders drawn away from the ears.

4. Lean back slightly, keeping your knees bent.

5. Lift your legs off the floor, until your shins are parallel to the floor.

6. Spine is straight.

7. Arms are straight.

8. For more challenge, try straightening your legs. Focus on your core strength.

9. Hold here for 3–10 breaths. Rest and repeat 3–5 times. You may be surprised how long you can maintain this posture. *You are stronger than you think.*

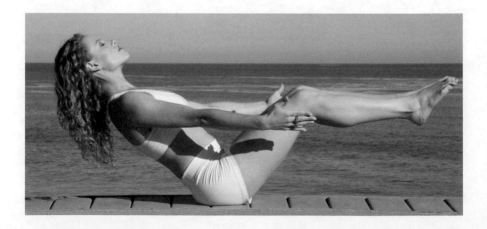

हेअर्त्ओपेनेर्स्अन्द्बच्क्बेन्द्स्

HEART-OPENERS AND BACKBENDS

Ustrasana (Camel Pose)

1. Kneel on the floor with your shins hips distance apart and parallel.

2. Place the palms of your hands on the lower back or upper buttocks, fingers point down.

3. Lightly, carefully, mindfully reach your hands behind you toward your heels, opening the front side of your body. Lift belly in and up, drop tailbone down toward the floor.

4. Elbows squeeze together opening your heart.

5. Let go in the shoulders.

6. Allow the head and neck to relax backward.

7. Stay here 5–15 breaths.

To release, come back up standing on the shins. Sit back on your heels, and bring the palms together at your heart. Pause. Repeat up to 3 times.

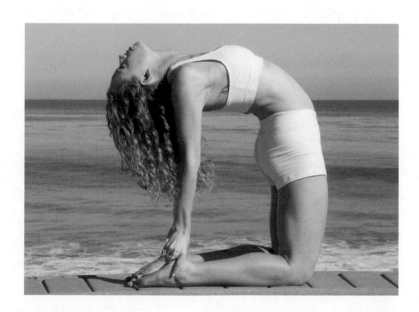

Setu Bandhasana (Bridge Pose)

Bridge Pose stimulates the adrenals glands, opens the lungs, is invigorating and good for depression.

1. Lie flat on your back with your arms at your sides.

2. Bend your knees, planting your feet into the ground—they are hip-distance and parallel.

3. Press down the inner edges of your feet to lift your hips.

4. Lift your hips toward the sky.

5. Arms stay extended down by your sides, or you may want to clasp your hands in order to open your shoulders and roll the chest open.

6. Slightly draw the belly in; extend the tailbone toward the heels,

7. stabilizing the lower back and opening the heart. Be sure to keep the thighs drawing in and parallel for safety, the knees stacking over the heels.

8. Hold here for 5–15 breaths.

9. Gently roll yourself down to the ground vertebra by vertebra.

10. Rest—place the hands on the belly, keeping a neutral spine. Repeat this pose up to three times. Once you are complete with all of your backbends, you may bring your knees into the chest.

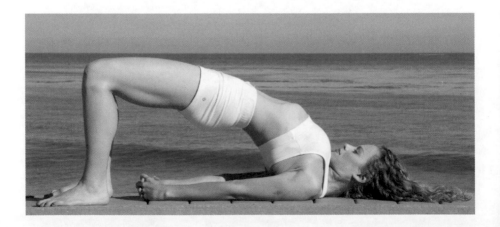

Urdhva Dhanurasana (Upward Bow/Wheel Pose)

1. Lie on your back.

2. Bring your heels close to your body.

3. Bend your elbows, bringing the palms of your hands, under your shoulders. Fingers point toward your feet.

4. On an inhale, press your palms into the floor as you lift your hips into the air. (Elbows need to stay in on the ride up.) This is really hard but it protects your shoulders, which can probably use a break—they've been carrying around enough, haven't they?

5. Straighten your arms as you lift your head off the floor—be careful not to lock out your elbows!

6. The knees should not splay out; remain parallel.

7. Breathe here for 5–15 breaths.

8. On an exhale, tuck your chin into your chest. Roll down carefully, one vertebra at a time.

9. Rest.

10. Once you are complete with all of your backbends, you may bring your knees into the chest.

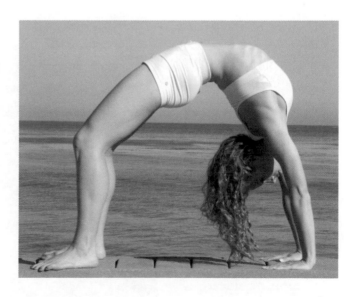

तइस्त्स्

TWISTS & FOLDS—LETTING GO

Ardha Matsyendrasana (Half Lord of the Fishes Pose)

1. Sit on the floor with your legs straight in front of you.

2. Bend your knees toward the sky. Both feet on the floor.

3. Slide your left foot under your right leg to the outside of your right hip.

4. The outside of the left leg lays on the floor.

5. Step the right foot to the floor on the outside of the left leg.

6. The right knee will point to the sky.

7. Exhale, twisting your body toward the inside of the right thigh.

8. Right palm presses into the floor, down and away to create a rise in the heart.

9. Feel your whole body twisting and detoxifying, letting go of anything that no longer serves. On the inhale, elongate the spine. On the exhale, twist deeper.

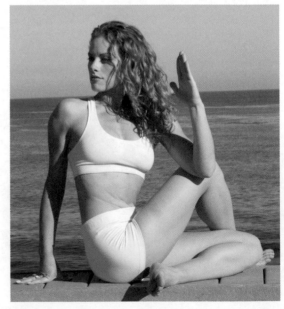

10. Hold this pose for 5–15 breaths .

11. Release slowly and repeat on side 2.

Dandasana (Staff Pose)

1. Sit with the legs straight out in front of you on the floor.

2. The legs are together. Roll the thighs in, until the inner edges of the feet come together.

3. Allow the arms to rest along the side body with the palms resting on the mat.

4. Activate the leg muscles by pressing out through the ball of the foot.

5. Ground the legs into the floor strongly—don't lock your knees!

6. Lift the heart toward the sky. Feel the collarbones spread open. Allow the shoulder blades to actively drop back and down.

7. Lengthen through the crown of the head up toward the sky.

8. Root the sitbones down into the ground.

9. Stay here for 5–15 breaths.

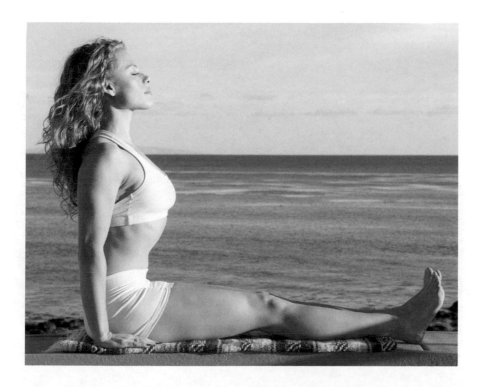

Janushirasana (Seated Forward Fold)

1. Sit up straight with your legs together, stretched out in front.

2. Flex both feet.

3. Inhale, and stretch your arms up over your head, while lengthening the entire spine upward.

4. Exhale and fold forward down over your legs.

5. If you are able, grab your feet. If not, just rest your hand on top of your shins.

6. Maintain integrity in the straight spine .

7. Relax your body into a luxurious hold.

8. Hold for 5–15 breaths, or set a timer and hold for 3–15 minutes.

Ahhhhhh . . .

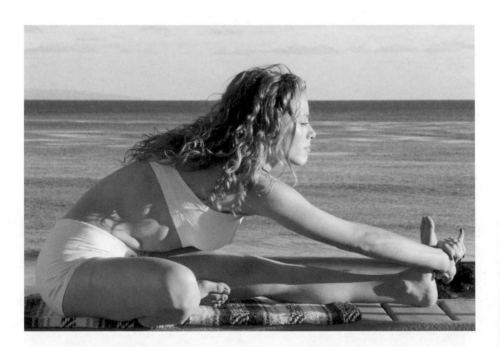

हपि्ओपेने्रस्

HIP OPENER (RELEASING EMOTION)

Eka Pada Rajakapotasana Variation (Thread the Needle Pose)

1. Lay on your back, knees bent, feet are hips distance apart.

2. Cross your right ankle over your left thigh.

3. Flex your right foot.

4. Clasp your hands around your left thigh and lightly pull your left thigh toward the trunk of your body.

5. Find your own sweet spot where the pleasure meets the pain and feel a release at that edge (likely somewhere in your hip/butt area).

5. Hold for 5–15 breaths. Ahhh . . .

6. We hold much emotional tension in our hips, so this is an excellent pose for moving through the challenging emotions of a break-up or grief. It's amazing what "old stuff" you may discover hiding out in there.

7. Breathe here for at least one minute. Don't forget to exhale!

8. Switch sides.

9. Repeat on Side 2.

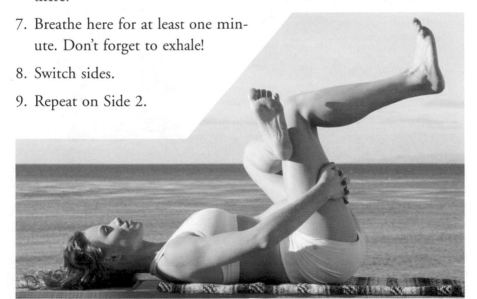

रेस्तोरतविइन्वेर्सओिन्स्

RESTORATIVES & INVERSIONS

Viparita Karani (Legs Up the Wall Variation)

1. Sit with your bottom next to the wall.

2. In one swift movement, swing both legs up on to the wall.

3. Scoot your bottom in toward the wall, as your legs find length.

4. Allow your spine to lengthen against the floor, finding support.

5. Stay in this position for 1–15 minutes.

6. Enjoy the restorative effects of this relaxing pose. During times of pain, grief, or even just stress, restorative poses have the power to recharge your physical body. Enjoy this time, and take care of yourself.

7. To exit, bend your knees into your chest and lightly rock to your right side.

8. Take a beat there, before rising into a seated position.

9. Breathe!

Supta Baddha Konasana
(Reclined Bound Angle Pose)

1. Come onto your back, bringing the knees into your chest.

2. Bring the soles of your feet together, allowing the knees to gently drape toward the floor.

3. In this Heartbreak Yoga variation, we will put one hand on the heart center and one hand on the low belly.

4. One hand is on the Anahata (heart) Chakra and one is on the Manipura (third) Chakra, activating your sense of strength, will, grit and power.

5. Feel your breath coming in and out of the body

6. Allow for any feelings that may come up. Take this moment to let your physical, subtle and energetic bodies heal.

7. Enjoy this relaxed pose for one to fifteen minutes.

8. To exit, place the hands on the outsides of the thighs, gently guiding them toward each other. Bring the knees into the chest. Hug them into your body. Take a full deep breath, and then slowly roll to one side. Take a beat, and then carefully move into a comfortable cross-legged seated position.

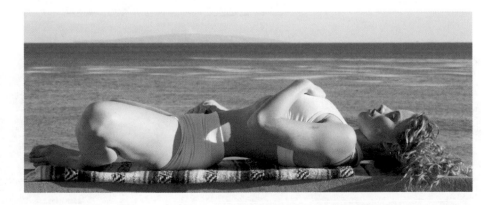

Savasana

1. Lie down on your mat with a flat back.

2. Extend your arms and legs, letting your feet flop open.

3. Find length through the bottoms of your feet.

4. Palms face up in an open receptive position, fingers relaxed.

5. Feel an opening and spreading in the collarbones.

6. Allow the shoulders to settle into the floor.

7. Let your eyes close and find a soft gaze within down, toward the heart.

8. Feel the base of your tongue relaxing.

9. Allow the lips to release.

10. Let go of any holding in the eyes, jaw, temple.

11. Scan your body from the crown of your head the soles of your feet. Is there anywhere you can let go, heal, or love a little bit more?

12. Take several deep breaths into your low belly (if you are using the ujjayi breath, let it go now).

13. Stay in this position for 1–15 minutes.

Please do NOT skip this pose. That's like writing an entire term paper in a Word doc and forgetting to press "save." There's really just no point.

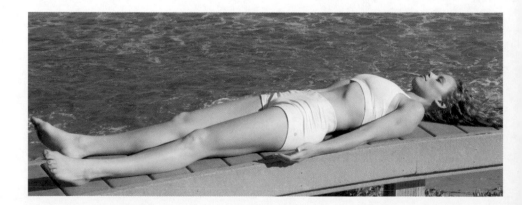

When you are ready to exit, wiggle the fingers and toes slightly, hug your knees into your chest releasing any last bit of tension. Roll to one side and find a comfortable cross-legged seated position.

You may want to close out your practice with an "Aum" or the prayer "Lokah Samastah Sukhino Bhavantu." (May all Beings everywhere be happy, safe and free.)

हेअलनिग्अब्रोकेन्हेअर्त्

10 MINUTE MEDITATION
FOR HEALING A BROKEN HEART

RECOMMENDED TOOLS: Stopwatch or cellphone alarm clock

Can be done anytime—recommended first thing in the morning and last thing before bed (if possible).

1. Take a comfortable cross-legged seated position (Sukasana or Padmasana), sit upright in a chair, or lay on your back. Be mindful that your spine is straight.

2. Rest your hands on top of heart (like a two-handed pledge of allegiance).

3. Breathe in. Focus your attention on the breath coming into your body, expanding your abdomen and lungs.

4. Breathe out. Place your attention on your abdomen and lungs letting go.

5. Continue this for five full breath cycles. Allow the breath to move in and out of the body at its own rhythm. You don't need to control or contort the breath, it knows what to do (it does it when we're sleeping, after all).

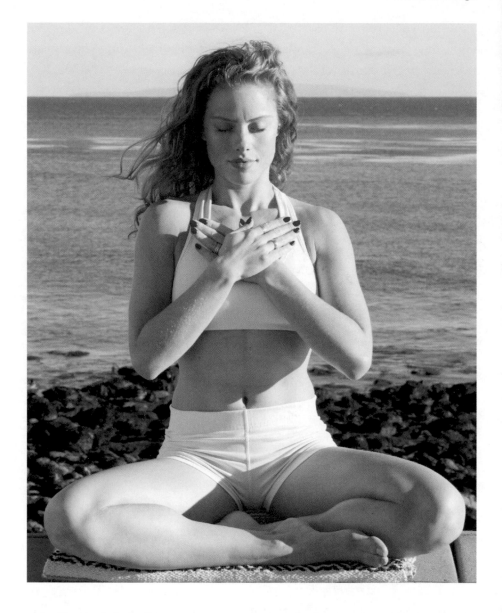

6. On an inhale focus your attention to the heart center. See it in your mind's eye. What does it look like? What does it feel like?

7. On the exhale, focus your attention on the heart center. What does it look like? What does it feel like?

8. Breathe in and out of the heart center for eight full breath cycles.

9. Now . . . with attuned awareness to the subtle messages of the body, feel the physical, emotional and energetic pains of heartbreak. Does your heart feel heavy? Are you nauseated? Does your body ache? Are you lethargic? Does your jaw feel rigid? Is the pain a color? Is it a shape? How would you describe it to a trusted friend? Is it felt somewhere specific? Can you locate where the grief is living?

   (If you cannot physically find it, but you know it's lurking around, you may want to ask yourself "Where am I holding my pain?" "What do I need to know about this pain?")

10. Once you have located the hurt, start to approach it with your breath. *You are braver than you think.* Take a deep breath in to the pain. See your breath filling the pain, feel the breath creeping into every corner of the pain. As is necessary breathe out. On the next inhale, repeat. Breathe into the pain center again.

11. How does the breath penetrate the pain? Perhaps your breath is able to make the consistency of the pain less dense, dark, deep or heavy? Perhaps you are able to stretch it apart, or make it more transparent. Continue to breathe in and out of the pain for ten full breaths. Is there anything it wants to tell you? Is there anything you need to know?

12. Is your breath able to open, lighten or remove any pain? On your next inhale, ask the pain to move with you to your heart center. Place the pain right there in your heart. It may feel unbearable for a moment, but you can do this. *Your heart is stronger than you think.*

13. Feel the pain in your heart totally and completely. Does it feel like a big crack? Is it an unimaginable weight? *You are brave. You can do this.* Breathe into the pain. Know that the heart is the strongest, most dynamic force in all of existence. Within your heart is the innate wisdom of every cell in your body, the knowledge of all the stars in the sky and the support of all consciousness. Your heart has the power to transform, and transmute this pain.

14. Breathe into this pain as high, wide, and large as you can.

15. As you breathe out, feel the pain leaving your heart center, know that your very intention, your own power within, can alleviate this suffering. It may not happen today or tomorrow, but the ache will leave you.

16. Breathe into the pain deeply, fully, with every ounce of energy you have.

17. As you breathe out, watch it leaving your body; breathe it out.

18. Using your stopwatch or cellphone alarm, continue this for five minutes; Breathing in healing, breathing out pain. You may want to say to yourself, I breathe in peace, I breathe out pain. I breathe in love, I breathe out separation. I breathe in healing, I breathe out sorrow. Whatever words resonate with you.

19. At the conclusion of the five minutes, feel the heart center. Thank it for all it has done today. Now, set your alarm for three minutes. Breathe the sensation of love into your heart center. Feel it filling your heart fully. Does love feel warm? Is it comforting? Is this feeling of breath entering your heart nourishing to the muscles? Can you feel the heart chakra shining? Perhaps it is like a little shower of sunshine, or wind. Continue to breathe into the heart center, watching the love expand from your heart into the room you are sitting in, into the street where you live, down the roads, into the city, the field, the ocean, just watch your love pouring out over everything into the universe. Know that you have the support of all of creation here to help in your healing.

20. At the end of the three minutes, feel your hands on your heart center. Does anything feel different? Slowly bring your awareness back to the physical body, back to the room. As you are ready slowly open your eyes.

21. If you have done this meditation first thing in the morning, set an intention for your day "I will be kind to myself." "I will see love wherever I go." "I will focus on healing today."

22. If you have done this meditation before bed, you may want to ask yourself "Is there anything I need to know while I sleep?" "Is there anything for me to learn?" You may be surprised at how quickly the answers come to a mind and heart at rest.

You may want to close out the practice with an "Aum," or a prayer for peace: *Lokah Samastah Sukhino Bhavantu.* ("May all Beings everywhere be happy, safe and free.") You may like to say it once, three times, for several minutes hours, or even days.

मेदतितिओन् ओर् अहेअर्त् अत् पेअचे

MEDITATION FOR A HEART AT PEACE

RECOMMENDED TOOLS: Stopwatch or cellphone alarm clock

1. Come into a comfortable cross-legged seated position (Sukhasana or Padmasana) or sit upright in a chair with your feet on the floor.

2. Set your alarm for 5, 10, 20, or 30 minutes.

3. Place your palms facing up on your knees (or thighs) in Jnana Mudra (thumb and index finger touching in the "okay" symbol). Jnana means "wisdom," Mudra means "seal." Also known as a sign language to the Gods—a direct message requesting universal knowledge. When we are in Jnana Mudra , we are asking for wisdom or guidance.

4. Root your sit bones into the ground, be sure the spine is aligned, let your chin drop slightly, allowing the neck to lengthen.

5. Beginning at the crown of your head, scan your body for any tension you can let go of.

6. Bring your awareness to the heart center.

7. Breathe into the heart center. (Remember when we learned to breathe into the low belly allowing the breath to cascade in and out of the body, letting go of any tensions?)

8. Ask your heart "Is there anything I need to know?" "Is there anything you want to teach me?" "Is there anything I can let go of?"

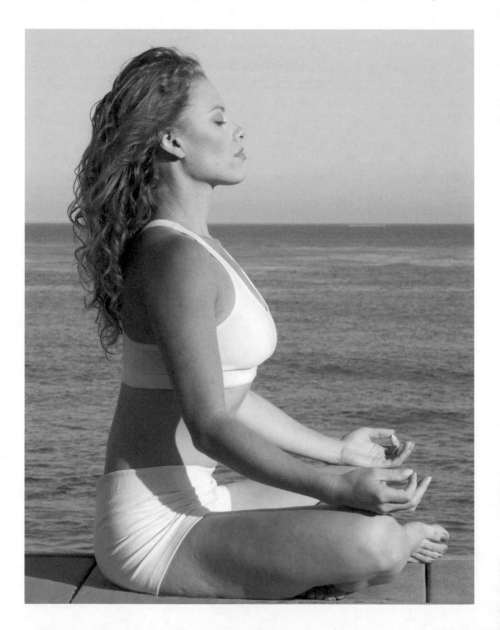

"Is there anything I'm holding in my heart I don't need to carry anymore?"

9. Sit silently and wait for the answers to reveal themselves. It may be today, it may tomorrow, it may be next week, next month, but if you stay quiet, you will get answers. Continue this practice for 5, 10, 20, 30 minutes—as long as you like.

10. At the conclusion of this practice, be sure to thank your inner guidance, the guidance from within, above, wherever you feel it comes from.

You may want to seal the practice with an "Aum" or "Lokah Samastah Sukhino Bhavantu," or simply bow your head in gratitude.

हेअर्त्सोन्ग्मेदतितिओन्

HEART SONG MEDITATION

RECOMMENDED TOOLS: Stopwatch or cellphone alarm clock

1. Come into a comfortable cross-legged seated position (Sukhasana or Padmasana) or sit upright in a chair with your feet on the floor.

2. Set your alarm for 5, 10, 20 or 30 minutes.

3. Place your palms together at your heart in Anjali Mudra (prayer position).

4. Root your sit bones into the ground; be sure the spine is aligned. Let your chin drop slightly allowing the neck to lengthen.

5. Beginning at the crown of your head, scan your body for any tension you can let go of.

6. Bring your awareness to the heart center.

7. On an inhale feel the breath filling your lower belly, on the exhale begin to chant "Aum" into your heart center.

8. On the next inhale feel the clear, clean, healthy air filling your body with fresh, positive prana (life-force energy).

9. On the exhale, chant "Aum" into your heart center.

10. When we chant "Aum" we are aligning ourselves with all of creation. We attune to the frequency of the universe. We ask for the knowledge of all life.

11. Allow the vibration to penetrate your heart center.

12. Feel the "Aum" growing from the heart, throughout the entire body.

13. As "Aum" widens out into the gross and subtle body, allow it to wash away any feelings of stuck, stagnant, tensions. Let it clear off anything you don't need anymore. Allow the sound to take with it any tensions or sadness that are no longer serving you.

14. If an emotion arises that is more subtle, allow the "Aum" to open and widen it. Ask the emotion what it is there to teach you, or simply allow it to fade away.

15. Continue this for 5, 10, 20, 30 minutes.

To seal the practice you may want to bow your head in gratitude for the healing you have requested.

"May today there be peace within. May you trust that you are exactly where you are meant to be. May you use those gifts that you have received, and pass on the love that has been given to you. May you be content knowing you are a child of God. Let this presence settle into your bones, and allow your soul the freedom to sing, dance, praise and love. It is there for each and every one of us."

—St. Thérèse de Lisieux

YOGA NIDRA

Common complaints of heartbreak include "Can't eat, can't sleep, can't breathe." The practice of Yoga Nidra addresses the "Can't sleep" symptom. It is the yogic prescription for cardiac patients and those recovering from grief and trauma. This practice is known to unburden the heart of underlying mental and emotional tensions that reside in the physical and subtle bodies. Mindful yoga asana teacher Maggie Mellor explains:

> *"The practice of yoga nidra allows entry into the deepest level of Being. This is the place of truth. Anyone with trauma can experience this and feel perfectly at peace. Suffering is not suppressed but integrated into the Being. The story, the personal circumstance, the particular form of suffering falls away at this time. How helpful to know that there is a place within that is always at rest and totally okay!"*

To practice yoga nidra just get into bed—what else are you doing before going to sleep? C'mon, give it a try.

Lay down on your back. Be sure your head and neck are in a straight line to support the spine. Palms face up. Let your body sink into the bed. Settle and relax. There is nothing you need to do right now, nowhere you need to go, nothing you need to think. You are about to travel into a peaceful place inside of yourself. Breathe deeply, allowing the day to begin to melt away.

Know that you are held in this safe space. No one is going to hurt you here; you are safe. It is okay to let go of some of the edges, and come into a place of stillness.

Once you are still, feel your body getting heavy. Feel yourself sinking into the bed, letting go of any held tensions or anxieties—no longer needed.

Take five deep breaths in and out of the low belly, allowing for deep relaxation and nourishment.

Feel the mind start to slow. Let the chatter fade away. Breathe deep.

On the next breath set your sankalpa, your intention. Is your heart longing for healing? Is your mind longing for peace? What is your soul crying for? Create a short affirmative sentence, such as "I am at peace," "I am healed," "I am okay." Whatever you choose will be right for you today. *Your heart always knows.*

Mentally state your sankalpa three times. The resolve made during yoga nidra is planted deep within the subconscious mind.

We will begin rotation of consciousness scanning the body, letting go of any physical holds that are no longer needed.

Place your attention on the right thumb, let go of any tension you feel there. You may feel a subtle healing energy, nourishing your physical body. Let go of any holding, stress, or tension.

Now move your attention to the first finger of the right hand, then the middle finger, the ring finger and to your little finger.

Bring your attention to the palm of your right hand . . .

1. Wrist	8. Hip and waist	14. Bottom of the right foot
2. Forearm	9. Thigh	
3. Elbow	10. Knee	15. Big toe
4. Upper arm	11. Shin and calf muscle	16. Second toe
5. Right shoulder		17. Third toe
6. Armpit	12. Ankle	18. Fourth toe
7. Side of the chest	13. Heel	19. Little toe

Now bring your awareness to the left hand . . .

1. Thumb	10. Upper Arm	18. Ankle
2. Index finger	11. Left Shoulder	19. Heel
3. Middle finger	12. Armpit	20. Bottom of the left foot
4. Ring finger	13. Side of the chest	
5. Little finger	14. Hip and waist	21. Left big toe
6. Palm	15. Thigh	22. Second toe
7. Wrist	16. Knee	23. Third toe
8. Forearm	17. Shin and calf muscle	24. Fourth toe
9. Elbow		25. Little toe

Breathing

1. Right buttock	4. Right middle back	6. Right upper back
2. Right lower back	5. Left middle back	7. Left upper back
3. Left lower back		

8. Right shoulder blade
9. Left shoulder blade
10. Spinal cord (from top to bottom and back again)
11. Back of the neck
12. Back of the head
13. Top of the head
14. Forehead
15. Right Eyebrow
16. Left Eyebrow
17. Eyebrow center (Breathe into it three times)
18. Right Eye
19. Left Eye
20. Both Eyes

21. Right Ear
22. Left Ear
23. Right Cheek
24. Left Cheek
25. Right Nostril
26. Left Nostril
27. Tip of the nose
28. Upper lip
29. Lower lip
30. Teeth
31. Gums
32. Tongue
33. Lower Jaw
34. Throat
35. Neck
36. Right Collarbone
37. Left Collarbone
38. Right Chest
39. Left Chest

40. Heart Center (Breathe into it three times)
41. Upper Abdomen
42. Lower Abdomen
43. Navel center
44. Whole right leg
45. Whole left leg
46. Both legs together
47. Whole right arm
48. Whole left arm
49. Both arms together
50. Whole right side of your body
51. Whole left side of the body
52. Whole physical body (breathe into it three times)

Become aware of your whole physical body from the crown of your head all the way to the soles of your feet. Breathe into your whole physical body. Be sure to include the right side, the left side, the front side, the back side, breathe deeply and fully into your entire body, feeling awareness of each part of your body at once. Feel your focus nourishing and vitalizing each cell of your body.

Continue to breathe deeply, feel a sense of peace. Remain quiet and still. Feel whole and complete. Know you have the power to heal yourself.

Rest here peacefully or relax into sleep.

If you are rising, wiggle the fingers and toes. Slowly roll to your right side and move into a seated posture. Seal out the practice with a prayer, and "Aum" or a few minutes of silence. Feel the deep relaxation and restoration you have just created within yourself.

Ahhhhhhhhh . . .

"Your task is not to seek for love,
but merely to seek and find
all the barriers within yourself
you have built against it."

—Rumi

CHAPTER 9

Healing

"I think that we have underestimated profoundly the human spirit and I feel that a peaceful and present individual can in the midst of great suffering bring about a quality of wisdom which is inherent to every individual."

—JOAN HALIFAX, PH.D., ZEN BUDDHIST ROSHI,
CAREGIVER FOR THE DYING

IN 1917 SIGMUND FREUD, KNOWN AS THE FATHER of psychoanalysis, wrote a whirlwind paper about grief called "Mourning and Melancholia." Freud observes:

Mourning

"Mourning is regularly the reaction to the loss of a loved person, or to the loss of some abstraction which has taken the place of one, such as one's country, liberty, an ideal, and so on."

Melancholy

"The distinguishing mental features of melancholia are a profoundly painful dejection, cessation of interest in the outside world, loss of the capacity to love, inhibition of all activity, and a lowering of the self-regarding feelings to a degree that finds utterance in self-reproaches and self-revilings, and culminates in a delusional expectation of punishment. This picture becomes a little more intelligible when we consider that, with one exception, the same traits are met with in mourning."

Mourning and Melancholia

"The disturbance of self-regard is absent in mourning; but otherwise the features are the same. Profound mourning, the reaction to the loss of someone who is loved, contains the same painful frame of mind, the same loss of interest in the outside world—in so far as it does not recall him—the same loss of capacity to adopt any new object of love (which would mean replacing him) and the same turning away from any activity that is not connected with thoughts of him. It is easy to see that this inhibition and circumscription of the ego is the expression of an exclusive devotion to mourning which leaves nothing over for other purposes or other interests. It is really only because we know so well how to explain it that this attitude does not seem to us pathological."

If you are experiencing that clinical loss of interest in the outside world, a prescription from grief counselors is to "Bear Witness," a practice in which you tell *your* truth. In the 90s, brave beauties Alanis Morissette and Gwen Stefani bled out into recording booths, allowing a combined 49 million listeners to bear witness to their betrayal. Writing about the rollercoaster ride of romantic relationships, Alanis's album *Jagged Little Pill* and Gwen Stefani's songs on the No Doubt album, *Tragic Kingdom* gave a new pack of pre-teen girls permission to feel their own pain.

While processing *Melancholy and The Infinite Sadness,* here are some questions worth asking yourself, answering aloud to another, or in a notebook somewhere:

1. Can you tell me in detail about this experience?

2. What about this makes sense?

3. What about this did not make sense?

4. Was there any part of this that surprised you?

5. Was there any part of this that didn't surprise you?

6. Did anything about this scare you?

7. Did anything about this make you feel safe or taken care of?

8. What were your greatest strengths in this scenario?

9. Do you have any weaknesses here, or things you wish you had done differently?

10. Do you really believe that would have changed the outcome?

11. Is there anything you can do to change that now?

12. Are you willing to accept what you can and cannot change?

13. Is there anything you can let go of here?

14. Where do you see yourself in this story?

15. Where do you see the others in this story?

16. Where do others see you in this story?

17. Is there anything you need from them to feel complete?

18. Is there anything they need from you to feel complete?

19. How are you different after this has happened?

20. Is there anything you have left out? Any last detail you may have forgotten?

21. What do you think you would need to feel safe to move on from this?

22. Are you able to attain that yourself, or do you need help?

23. Who is someone you can ask to help you?

24. Are you willing to do something today to move toward healing?

25. Are you complete?

A historically poignant portrait painted by this practice is deep within
the pages of *The Diary of Anne Frank*. During the Nazi occupation of
Germany, six million Jews were "exterminated." *While typing that word,
I just gagged. It's so disgusting I don't want it weighing down the pages of
this book. However, if I'm not brave enough to speak the truth and bear witness to this genocide, I have no right asking you to do the same with your
own personal tragedy. Trying again:* While Hitler reigned, six million Jews
were "exterminated." Anne Frank dreamt into her diary, and it is within
the pages of that cardboard-bound book we learned what coming of age
in the midst of war, hate, hope and fear could feel like. The Frank family, the van Daan family and an elderly, single dentist named Mr. Dus-
sel hid from Hitler's regime high above a warehouse in Amsterdam for
two full years.

This group experienced every essence of human emotion (including a
romantic subplot!). On September 3, 1944, the Nazis discovered the
secret annex and carted all eight off to internment camps. Anne Frank
was aboard a freight train taken to Auschwitz. An interviewed inmate
later recalls the conditions: Putrid food was served regularly, shouting
SS guards required scheduled showers, and the dead and dying simply
disappeared from the barracks. Completely decomposing physically,
mentally and emotionally, most inmates were almost able to ignore the
atrocities—walking ghosts awaiting the gas chamber, disconnected and
decayed. But Anne Frank never had that protective mechanism. She
couldn't block anything out. She cried into the eyes of naked gypsy girls
on their way to the crematory; she cried for Hungarian children who had
stood outside in the cold rain for nearly half a day awaiting their "exter-
mination"; and she cried for the family she feared had been "cleansed."

An excerpt from *The Diary of Anne Frank:*
Saturday, 20 June, 1942
  *I haven't written for a few days, because I wanted first of all to think
about my diary. It's an odd idea for someone like me to keep a diary, not
only because I have never done so before, but because it seems to me that
neither I—nor for that matter anyone else—will be interested in the unbo-*

somings of a thirteen-year-old schoolgirl. Still, what does that matter? I
want to write, but more than that, I want to bring out all kinds of things
that lie buried deep in my heart.

   There is a saying that "paper is more patient than the man," it came
back to me on one of my slightly melancholy days . . . I don't intend to
show this cardboard-covered notebook, bearing the proud name "diary" to
*anyone, unless I find a real friend, boy or girl, **probably nobody cares.***

PROBABLY NOBODY CARES?!

In 1945, just shy of 16 years old, Anne Frank died. Her diary has since sold more than 31 million copies and has been translated into 67 languages. It has been adapted for theatre, film, television and tolerance education curriculum.

Can you imagine a moment when this beautiful being whose surviving spirit has shed light on the world thought, "probably nobody cares"? If you think you don't matter, and love can't ever win, think of this strong little soul—and then think of the following:

I know someone whose grandparents *met in a concentration camp,* fell in love and later escaped that concentration camp. The extended family including children, grandchildren and great grandchildren now live in California's San Bernardino Valley. They gather each year for Yom Kippur. The day of atonement.

RESOURCES FOR HELP

If you feel yourself seriously slipping, please seek professional help. The following are some resources:

National Suicide Prevention Lifeline: 800-273-TALK (8255) • www.afsp.org

Crisis Helpline: 800-233-4357

Self-Injury: 800-366-8288

Al-Anon/Alateen: www.al-anon.alateen.org

DivorceCare: Divorce Recovery Support Groups: 919-562-2112

"There is beauty in suffering.
The rise greater than the fall.
Do you know you are a beautiful soul?"
—David Newman,
"Beautiful Soul/Om Namah Shivaya"

CHAPTER 10

Transition

*"Just when the caterpillar thought the world was over,
it became a butterfly."*

—Proverb

TRANSITION TAKES TIME.

Go easy on yourself.

In Charles Darwin's *Origin of the Species,* he speaks of evolution:

"We have seen that a species under new conditions of life may change its habits, or it may have diversified habits, with some very unlike those of its nearest congeners. Hence we can understand, bearing in mind that each organic being is trying to live wherever it can live . . . if we know of a long series of gradations in complexity, each good for its possessor, then under changing conditions of life, there is no logical impossibility in the acquirement of any conceivable degree of perfection."

The following are merely menu offerings for luxury cocoon living. Enjoy the metamorphosis. Soon you will soar, butterfly.

"Lovin', Touchin', Squeezin' "
—Journey

Sometimes when we're depressed or down, and it's difficult to even get out of bed, our bodies ache like we have the flu. Massage is one of the easiest, most luxurious ways to alleviate these subtle pains. It relaxes muscles (which release emotional stresses held in the body), it aids in digestion, improves circulation, and helps eliminate waste.

New York City's Bliss Spa lead masseuse, Ben Brown explains:

> *There are many schools of thought of how emotions affect the body, both positively and negatively. A simple example of how an emotion can affect the body is the physical action of frowning. When we're sad we frown, which requires more muscle contraction than smiling. The contracting muscles are holding tension, and long-term tension leads to pain. You can use this model of the frown and equate it to other parts of the body like the neck, shoulder or lower back or any area affected by emotional distress.*
>
> *Massage is helpful in releasing the "tense" area and thereby helping the body remove the physical pain of an emotion. The act of massage also releases endorphins, which create a natural high and reduce the levels of cortisol, the "stress" hormone. Small doses of cortisol can reduce pain sensitivity, while large doses causes these negative effects—lowered immunity and inflammatory responses in the body, decreased bone density, a decrease in muscle tissue and higher blood pressure to name a few.*

As we say in Santa Monica, "It's part of the practice." Go get a massage. You deserve it. I said so.

If that justification didn't work, try this one: Your body holds your heart, soul and mind. It is your tireless servant until the day you leave it. It's okay to treat it nicely.

Good? Are you making the appointment?

For daily care and maintenance of your body temple, certified massage therapist and kinesiologist Anne Olt advises self-massage:

"Self-massage is nurturing, especially if you have a broken heart; you don't need a lover's touch to feel good. You can nurture yourself. You can rub your own feet with oils and lotions."

Anne believed in this philosophy so strongly that she began a long career with Desert Essence. Her #1 recommended product is Jojoba Oil.

"Jojoba is a miracle oil, which is how Dessert Essence started—with that one product. The whole company was founded on jojoba oil in 1978 by Sridhar Silberfein, actually. Jojoba oil is actually a wax ester and it has almost the same molecular structure as the sebum [natural oil] our bodies produce; it's just one molecule off. It doesn't clog pours, so it's non-comedogenic. It has so many uses—for massage, dry skin, cuticles, you can use it to moisturize your scalp, you can put it on the ends of your hair overnight and wash it out. People even cleanse and use it as makeup remover because it's so good for your skin. It has been our number-one seller every year for almost 35 years now. It's not cut with anything. It's cold pressed, which means it's like olive oil—it is the mechanical extraction, and isn't heated over 120 degrees. We even have a USDA Organic and a 100% pure. Jojoba oil is also good for Celiacs (people who are allergic to wheat), as all of our organic lotions are wheat and gluten-free, as well as vegan. Some people are so sensitive that jojoba oil is all that their bodies respond positively to. It's nature's moisturizer. The Native Americans have been using it forever."

If oiling up isn't for you, any lotion is great for lube. Desert Essence Bulgarian Lavender and Coconut hand and body lotions are among my faves.

Give love (or at least oil and lotion) to every inch between. Your epidermis is your largest organ; therefore, it absorbs and processes more chemicals than its organ friends like the liver or kidneys. All your organs want to be fed yummy nourishing foods. For the epidermis, that is a diet of organic oils and lotions.

HOW TO SELF-MASSAGE

Neck and Shoulders

The cause of the ol' "pain in the neck" is most often attributed to the trapezius muscle—the one that holds all the tension and makes you look like a turtle if unattended.

1. With your right hand, locate the left trapezius muscle.

2. Beginning at the base of the neck, use a consistent rhythmic method to knead into the tension-trapped area moving out toward the arm.

3. Switch arms/sides.

4. Breathe deep!

Feet

1. Hold your right foot in your left hand.

2. Use your thumb to knead into the bottom of your foot moving out toward the toes and back toward the heel.

3. Gently, but firmly pull and stretch each toe.

4. Maintain rotation in your ankles by doing ankle circles in each direction.

"It Must Have Been the Roses"

—THE GRATEFUL DEAD

Can you recall the smell of home baked cookies? Christmas Trees? Jasmine? Fresh cut grass? Did you know our olfactory sense is the one most closely linked to our emotions? A great way to nurture and care for your sense of smell (and the emotions it's linked to) is by using essential oils. An essential oil is a highly concentrated, aromatic essence.

Elizabeth Golden, aromatherapist and founder of Golden Earth, explains:

"When I went to aromatherapy school I realized how valuable essential oils are, and that a lot of people didn't know about them. I wanted to create something that would be beneficial healthy, non-toxic and from nature. That is exactly what essential oils are. They all have healing properties. They are uplifting—they create a positive energy in your life. Just smelling an essential oil is a gift from Mother Earth. It's something you have to try. [She laughs.] The words don't really describe how great they make you feel. They are wonderful healers."

During the first phase of heartbreak, while you need some TLC, I recommend lavender. Its number one property is healing. In addition, it is known to calm, sooth, normalize, balance and relax. I have a friend who fell for lavender and its healing properties so hard during his divorce that he now sells it on the weekends at our local farmers' market. Talk about believing in the product! If you are lucky enough to have a farmers' market near you, check for this magic plant. If that is not an option, many health food stores carry essential lavender water, sprays, perfumes, massage oils, sachets and lotions. My favorite of these products is Aura Cacia Rollerball. You can roll a little dollop right under your nose, or on your upper lip to create a sense of calm. If you have ever sat in Los Angeles rush hour traffic, or been in the New York City subway when "a passenger has become ill" or the train gets stuck between stations, you can benefit from this product.

I love it so much I asked Aura Cacia and their parent company, Frontier Natural Brands, about the science behind the relief. Tom Havran, Aroma Therapy Product Developer, responded:

"Lavender oil consists of a remarkably high percentage of the ester compounds linalool and linalyl acetate in ratios approaching 40–45% of the total oil. These esters have a very light molecular weight in the realm of pheromones, so this may explain their powerful olfactory benefits and healing influence on a broken heart center. The soft, non-cloying floral aroma of lavender has a subtle and soothing effect on our emotions. The distinct and refreshing herbal undertone that lavender oil has counter-balances the floral notes to produce an overall harmonizing influence on the emotions.

It's interesting to note the color association of the violet flowers and green leaves of the plant to the violet color of the third eye chakra and the green color of the heart chakra. An enhancement of third eye insight (the lavender-colored chakra!) coupled with heart-centered compassion and understanding are the energy forces needed for recovery from a broken heart."

The fragrance we associate with opening and protecting the Anahata chakra is rose oil. It has the highest vibration of all the essential oils. The distillation process is a lot like the process of making wines from grapes— using 60,000 roses to make one ounce of rose oil. What a gift!

Elizabeth Golden of Golden Earth continues:

"Rose is a magnificent oil for just about anything, especially heartbreak; it really encompasses love—just unconditional love."

When it's time to get back into the groove and you need a boost, citrus can be a wonderfully awakening scent. I like using Burt's Bees Beeswax Lip Glosses. Many of them contain eucalyptus and/or mint, guaranteed to put a little pep in your step!

"The Revolution Will Not Be Televised"
—Gil Scott Heron

We are so over jammed with noise in the West: Cell phones, texting, emailing, Facebook, Pandora, TV, Sirius radio, regular radio, Siri, Shazam, ads in the back of the cabs, ads flashing fear and amber on the highway, ads at grocery store checkout lines, guilting us into giving a dollar. There is so much static, it's no wonder we *spazz* out and yell back at the person talking on their phone, reading the trades, unconsciously merging into our lane.

Western World responsibilities can pull us in a hundred different directions until our energy is so scattered and fragmented we can't even define "multi-task" let alone be fooled into thinking we can do it, or should want to do it, or are virtuous if we have done it. *"Hey asshole, that was my parking spot. See the blinker! I was here first, Bucko. I'll lay on this horn all day. Don't think I won't. Oh—sorry sir, I didn't realize that was you. So . . . about my six-month review that was scheduled for today, I, um, can I get you a cup of coffee?"*

Intentional mantra, meditation, and ambient music can make all the difference. It can call back the fragmented parts of yourself that were so busy multitasking you forgot you are a human being, not a human doing. We have limited time on the planet. Why waste it being spun out?

HEART-HEALING MUSIC

Here are some intentional heart-healing albums:

- *Heart Chakra Meditation*—Layne Redmond
- *Eternal Om*—Dick Sutphen
- *At Ease*—Various Artists
- *Illumination*—Steve Gorn, Ty Burhoe, Manose
- *Within*—Benjy Wertheimer and David Michael
- *The Spirit of Yoga*—Ben Leinbach
- *Savasana 2*—Wah!
- *Hangs with Angels*—Masood Ali Khan
- *Om Mani Padme Hum*—Budi Siebert

If you are chill-out curious but not ready to get your Enya on, Vitamin String Quartet and Vitamin Piano Series have now covered most of our favorite rock n' roll, punk and hip-hop tracks in mellow-friendly, peaceful pentameter.

Music industry and post-production sound veterans Michael and Jahna Perricone believed in this phenomenon so much they created the first online all conscious music download site, Omstream.com. There you will find a Heartbreak Yoga chill-out mix I made just for you!

"See Me, Feel Me"
—The Who

The Ancient Chinese Art of Feng Shui suggests that everything holds an energy. That energy is referred to as Chi (in Sanskrit we call it "Prana"— life force). Like wild women, this energy loves to run free and can't be broken. Chi's Personal Ad would look something like this: *Pulsating flow of life seeks clear paths. Turn-ons: Healthy, vibrant spaces, bodies and minds. Turnoffs: Microwaves, clutter, tense shoulders, self-defeating thoughts.*

Is your work and living space blossoming with the pregnant potential of pending love or is it a shrine to the "Say It Ain't So's"? The following are some additions guaranteed to raise the Love Vibe:

Flowers

Fresh flowers are chi and prana positive. Adding anything fresh, live and vibrant into your living space will raise the vibration. (Note: dead flowers are chi-negative. While we respect the cycle of life, we need also to respect our energetic space. Please dispose of the flowers as they die.

The Elements

The Ancient Greek, Empedocles, is the person believed to have created this term and its contents. To the Greeks, each sign of the zodiac, each human being, each home, each endeavor should contain all of the elements. They are defined as Earth, Air, Water and Fire. Are all of these represented in your living space?

Crystals

Crystals and gemstones are said to be from the earth, for the earth (sort of like those political campaigns "by the people, for the people"). Unlike election year promises, crystals always deliver the goods. They are known to contain mineral-based healing and guiding properties. While healing from heartbreak and opening the Anahata chakra, we are especially drawn to, and vibrating with, rose quartz. Its properties include releasing tension, stress and relieving symptoms of sadness and loneliness. Citrine is called upon to release fear. Carnelian promotes wisdom and helps to combat depression and lethargy. Red jasper is used to alleviate bereavement and fears around death (even of a relationship). If you are in need of one of these healing channels, the right one will likely find you. Keep your eyes open. ;)

Anahata Mandala

The word "mandala" is translated as "circle." These concentric diagrams are introduced in the Rig Veda, as having ritual and spiritual power. Aspirants use them as a visual point of focus for meditation and prayer. They organize the inner energies including the mental relationship to the ego. Famed psychologist Carl Jung regarded the mandala as a useful tool in individualization (moving into yourself and away from the collective unconscious).

The Mandala below was painted (and generously shared with us) by Paul Heusenstamm who clarifies, "The Mandala to me, more than any other teacher in this lifetime, has opened up a doorway into the symbolic language of the soul."

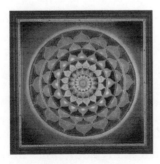

This mandala represents the Anahata Chakra.

"Crunchy Granola Suite"
—NEIL DIAMOND

Admit it. You want chocolate. I know, so do I. Humans have treated chocolate as an anti-depressant since the 12th century. The Aztecs practically worshipped it. Reason being, chocolate produces several chemical reactions in the brain known to lift spirits. Among them is the secretion of endorphins. Chocoholics receive an effect similar to a runner's high. Cocoa contains the neurotransmitter serotonin, the one that uncontrollably oozes when you fall in love, receive good news, or watch a funny movie. We get a high from the chemical compounds found in chocolate's caffeine as well—phenylethylamine and theobromine.

This is the first and last "way-left" liberal hippie health comment I will make, but I'm serious about it. Processed sugar is bad news. Do your homework on its health effects. Okay, I'm off the soapbox. For a yummy, not-so-lethal place to score your chocolate fix, try Fearless Chocolate—it's organic and fair trade!

Justin Schuster of Fearless Chocolate explains what it means to buy fair trade (conflict-free) chocolate (diamonds):

"Fearless Chocolate bars are crafted direct trade (that's one-step beyond fair trade) in collaboration with family-owned farms in Bahia, Brazil. By working with our farmers directly, we have unique access to cultivating each detail of our chocolate from farm to table. We collaborate with both the farm owners and farm labor to bring funding and delicious chocolate back into the local community. As we grow and develop, so too should the social and environmental conditions improve for the Bahian cocoa farmers we support. With each purchase we donate a "bite" of our chocolate back to promote community projects in Bahia as well as to customer-suggested changemakers."

Eat chocolate AND help people? Works for me!

There is no denying that in my household, the gateway drug of healthy eating was Amazing Grass's Chocolate. This is a super-easy way to get your daily dose of greens for the day.

Amazing Grass Company's CEO, Brandon Burt, explains how it actually can be easy to be *green:*

One of the reasons green super foods are so good for you is because it is really a foundation food that every single person should have more of in their body. Unfortunately, with today's fast-paced busy lifestyles and hectic schedules, we just don't have the time or wherewithal to get these great green foods in our diet. Days when you can sit down and prepare kale, spinach, broccoli and all these great meals, and eat all these great foods that you should be getting, just don't seem to happen. What we do is provide a very easy, convenient and affordable way to get an alkalizing, great source of vitamins, minerals and phytonutrients in your system. We do it with these dehydrated powders. They can be mixed in with your favorite beverage.

To give you just a little bit on the history side, these cereal grasses, which include wheatgrass, barley grass, oat grass and rye grass, grow into the grains you find in your morning cereal. Before they are a grain, they are a grass. Dr. Charles Schnabel in 1931 found that by putting these dehydrated cereal grasses in the chickens' feed, he was able to increase their egg production by about 250%. Back in the day, this was a huge story for anyone who was in the poultry, egg or farm business—getting that kind of an increase was just huge.

The key was, the grass had to be cut just before it jointed and grew into a full grain. They found that there were incredible benefits for people as well. In the 1930s and 1940s, they sold these cereal grass tablets. Doctors and pharmacists would recommend people take these greens, because they had such great nutrition. Even then they knew people weren't getting all the greens they could be getting!

Fast forward a little bit to the 1950s and you had these best-selling, "multivitamin" tablets. Then we, as a culture, started doing a lot of experimentation and we found that people could replicate some of these vitamins and minerals in a lab—then create Vitamin C in a lab, Vitamin A in a lab. When this One-A-Day multivitamin came out and now you could have all of these vitamins and minerals in this one little magic pill, people said, "Geez, I don't know if I need to take seven or eight of these wheatgrass tablets anymore when I can just get one little magic multivitamin and it's got one hundred percent of everything I need."

Fortunately, that pendulum is now swinging back the other way and people are realizing you can't really replicate Mother Nature by taking a little pill that has all of these synthetic, man-made vitamins in it. You just can't replicate all the co-factors and all the things that exist in Mother Nature. People are just starting to remember and understand that we need to eat these foods that have had thousands, if not millions, of years to develop and we need to be able to have these foods that are grown in the right climates.

It's unfortunate today that with a lot of produce, it's all about getting the biggest crop yield you can get, as fast as you can. Over the years our soil has been depleted. You're just not getting a lot of the vitamins and minerals you need in produce these days because of the fast growing cycles, because things can be picked way too early, etc. So, we go back to the old days. The cereal grasses, the greens that we grow, are planted in the fall and they grow through a cold winter to reach full nutritional potential.

Kansas, America's breadbasket, is the number one wheat-producing state because it has the ideal cold climate and the ideal healthy soil. The wheat has the ideal growing system. It roots down, pulls all the nutrients from the soil, and then in the spring when the sun comes out it starts to grow above the ground and just before it goes through that jointing process of going from a grass to a grain, we cut it right at its peak of nutrition. Then we dehydrate it at a low temperature, below 107 degrees. What that means is, we are protecting all the heat sensitive nutrients like enzymes and beta-carotene. We want to minimally process this. We want to keep everything that Mother Nature put in there.

It's not dissimilar to having the best leafy greens on Earth, like kale, collard greens and chard, and taking the moisture out of it. Those power greens are then pressed into a pellet to protect them from heat, light and oxygen, so it keeps everything really potent. We then mill them up into a fine powder, and that powder is then blended into our formulas. At the end of the day, when a consumer reaches for a bottle off the shelf or puts a scoop in their favorite drink, they are getting these incredible, rich, nutrient-dense greens that are super alkalizing. There is a lot of chlorophyll in there. You get the benefits of what Mother Nature created in a potent, easy, convenient way.

A lot of people find that when they consume the greens, this is something their body has been craving. It's alkaline. It's going to help keep the pH balance. Most of us today, with all the processed foods out there, stress and environmental factors, our pH balance is a little too much on the acidic side. By consuming alkalizing foods, like greens, you're helping to balance your body's pH, which in turn, helps your metabolism and helps you burn fat. When you are more acidic, your body has to store fat to protect your cells from the nature of your blood—your pH.

So, you get a lot of great benefits, not least of which is that you are helping to get your daily quota of green leafy vegetables. If you talk to any doctor, nutritionist or dietician, they are going to tell you that if you can get more servings of fruits and veggies in your diet every day, it's a good thing. Look at the stats—I think it's still up around 95 percent or higher—of people who just don't get enough servings a day. This provides a very easy, concentrated way to get those greens in your diet every day, and get what your body is craving and what it needs . . . every day.

We clean our homes, take out the trash, and make sure there isn't that little glob of toothpaste in the sink. While we are letting go physically and mentally, why not let go of some of the accumulated toxins in our bodies too? After time, preservatives from the foods we eat, the air we breathe and the products we use on our body and clothing can accumulate in our system. If we don't flush out this build up, it can turn into dis-ease.

We all know—more fruits and veggies, less take-out. At the risk of sounding like a character out of Neil Diamond's *Crunchy Granola Suite,* a green juice a day keeps the doctor away. If you are in a big city like LA or NYC, there are places to get FRESH green juices, fruit juices and smoothies.

- In NYC—The Juice Press
- In LA—Pressed Juicery
- In Between—Evolution Green Juice is available at many grocers.

  (Pressed Juicery & Blue Print Cleanse will ship anywhere in the U.S.!)

If you're not buying all this healthy green drink hootenanny, Jess Hilton N.C., HHC, Culinary Instructor and Celebrity Private Chef, has created Heartbreak Yoga Comfort Food just for us!

Chocolate Truffles (chocolate)

1 cup dates, pitted

$1/2$ cup almond meal (or any finely chopped nut)

$1/2$ cup Amazing Grass Chocolate Superfood
or Cocoa Powder

$1/4$ cup Cocoa Powder
or finely chopped almonds

In a large bowl, cover dates with boiling water and cover, until dates are softened. Reserve liquid and put dates in a food processor and purée.

Combine date purée with almond meal and Superfood. Stir to combine.

Scoop 1 tablespoon of mix and roll into a ball. Continue with the rest of the date, almond, Superfood mix. Drop each truffle into a bowl with the cocoa powder and toss until coated. Remove to a clean plate and refrigerate until firm.

Crispy Garbanzos (crispy)

2 cups cooked garbanzos
or 1 can, rinsed

2 tablespoons olive oil

1 tablespoon ground chipotle

1 cup salted pistachios

Toss garbanzos with 1 tablespoon olive oil and chipotle. Place on a baking sheet and place in 300-degree preheated oven for 15 minutes or until garbanzos are crispy.

While garbanzos are roasting, put the pistachios in the bowl used for garbanzos. Add garbanzos to the pistachios and toss. Taste for seasoning.

Kale Chips (crispy)

1 bunch kale, stems removed

2 tablespoons olive oil

Sea salt

Break the greens into smaller pieces, toss in a large bowl with a couple of tablespoons of olive oil and sprinkle with sea salt. You just want to lightly coat the leaves with the olive oil, not soak them with the oil. Lay them out flat on a baking sheet and bake in an oven preheated to 300 degrees until crispy. This takes about 10–20 minutes.

Rose-Scented Oatmeal (creamy)

$1/2$ cup steel cut oats

$1/2$ cup quinoa, rinsed

2 cups water

$1/2$ cup milk or nut milk

pinch salt

1 cactus pear, peeled (or mango)

$1/4$ cup hazelnuts

1–2 tablespoons honey (or to taste)

1 tablespoon rose water

Combine quinoa, oats, water and salt in a saucepan. Bring to a boil, cover and reduce to a simmer. Cook about 20 minutes or until most of the water is absorbed and grains are tender. Add milk to desired consistency and divide into two serving bowls.

While grains are cooking, coarsely chop hazelnuts and put in a bowl. Add rose water and honey, stir to combine.

Put pear in a blender to purée and then strain to remove the seeds. (If using mango, no need to strain).

To serve, swirl the pear purée into the grains and top with the nut mixture.

HEART HEALTHY FOODS

Acorn Squash	Dark chocolate	Soymilk
Almonds	Flaxseed	Spinach
Asparagus	Kidney Beans	Sweet potato
Black Beans	Oatmeal	Tea
Blueberries	Oranges	Tofu
Broccoli	Papaya	Tomatoes
Brown rice	Red bell peppers	Tuna
Cantaloupe	Salmon	Walnuts
Carrots		

Inspired by Jess's genius but feeling way lazy? Santa Monica's Rawvolution offers mailable, organic, all raw, weekly meal packages called "The Box." Hotties of all ages including Alicia Silverstone, Susan Sarandon and Cher all swear by them. An actor friend of mine exiled to the outskirts of rainy London may have only survived his long shoot-days and damp, two-banger trailer because of the joy that little weekly package provided him. Well that, and his subscription to Gaiam TV, but we'll learn more about that later.

For info on Rawvolution, The Box, The Pressed Juicery, and Amazing Grass, check out heartbreakyoga.com

Deede-ee deet deet deet deet deet deet deedle dee de . . .

"Don't Forget to Love Yourself."

—Soren Kierkegaard

AYURVEDA

I have doctor friends in Beverly Hills, Chicago, Miami and New York City. It would be a HIPAA violation for me to say much more, so come close and I'll whisper it . . . *90 percent of their patients are on an anti-depressant and sleeping pill of some kind.* Yup, that's right—90 percent. Then there's the obesity epidemic, and the number of people wearing pink in October in support of a loved one who has died from, or survived breast cancer. One in 88 babies is born with Autism, and 8.3 percent of the population has diabetes. That's an awful lot of sick for the "richest" country in the world's health "care" system, isn't it? Is anyone else alarmed that something might have gone awry somewhere?

Ayurveda is the Vedic health system of India dating back to 500 BCE. "Ayur" is translated to "Life" and "Veda" means "knowledge. This "Life Knowledge" addresses all aspects of health—mental, physical, emotional and spiritual.

Premal Patel, M.D. has a family medical practice in Texas. In addition, she studied at the Ayurvedic Institute with Dr. Vasant Lad. She currently serves as Wellness Director for Banyan Botanicals Ayurveda. I asked her to explain the Ayurvedic basics and best care for a broken heart. (Permission from your HMO, a referral from your primary care provider, pharmaceuticals and co-pay not required to read this.)

> Dr. Patel: In brief, Ayurveda is basically the traditional medical system that comes from the Vedic culture in India. There are two core principles of Ayurveda:
>
> 1. It looks at health as an integral connection of body, mind and spirit, so body mind and spirit are all integrally connected when it comes to health. One affects the other. So, to find health and wellbeing, you have to address body mind and emotions, which create spirit. All three have to be addressed when you want to find health.

2. When it comes to Ayurveda, the second part of that is every person is unique. Every person has a unique state of balance.

Poor health usually comes from each of us getting off of our unique
state of balance, so returning to good health is a unique and individual journey for each person. It looks different for each person, so what
it means for you to be healthy should never be determined by comparing to someone else.

As a tradition system of medicine, the very nature of Ayurveda is
to address the root of the issue. It doesn't just try to solve the surface
system. It really looks for the common underlying thread among everything that is showing up. It's the root imbalance. Ayurveda addresses the
root to then help all the symptoms that are appearing on the surface.

That root, again, addresses the whole person. People look at health
as a physical thing, but your physical health is never going to reach a
state of balance if your mind, your emotions and your spirit are off
balance. So to be really able to account for your entire being, is what
health means to me. You want to address your whole being.

Amy: What would be your Ayurvedic prescription to help aid in the
healing of heartbreak?

Dr. Patel: It's really of key importance to address your whole being,
but starting with some sort of yoga routine or pranayam (breathing)
routine. They are really going to address that sense of inner peace.
Often when we are facing heartbreak, when we are addressing the sadness, the grief, the anger, all those things, they're coming from us looking externally for love, for joy, for happiness and to find that sense of
peace and that happiness from within, there has to be some sort of
reflective meditative practice. So meditation along with yoga and
pranayam are key.

In terms of supplements, there are four herbs that come to mind
for me when we are talking about heartbreak, loss and grief.

1. **Arjuna** is a traditional remedy that is used to support the heart in
general. Ayurveda looks more at the subtle sides of the plants, not
just their bio-chemical nature. What's really neat about Arjuna refers
to the character in The Vedic Epic, The Mahabharata. Arjuna was

one of the great warriors in that. In the moment of battle on the battlefield, he forgot his true nature, his own inner nature and he forgot his dharma [Sanskrit word for destiny]. In doing that, he lost his courage. It was after reciting The Bhagavad Gita that he remembers those things, and he is able to find his courage. So the subtle nature of the herb Arjuna is really to regain that inner self confidence, that inner courage and that inner peace.

2. **Ashwagandha** has a dual nature to it, and is known as an adaptive. It brings a subtle sense of calm and it also energizes. When you are looking at the emotions of heartbreak—loneliness, sadness, grief— they have a vata (moving) component to them, that loneliness, separation and anxiety. They also may manifest as feelings of stress, just kind of rattled nerves, loss of sleep all those things. Ashwagandha is good to help calm that vata, to really rejuvenate the system to help with stress, sleep, the frazzled nerves and bring a sense of energy as well so that the lethargy and that dragging feeling can also be remedied.

3. **Guduchi:** If you look at the actual leaf, it's heart-shaped. It's an herb that for centuries has been known as a heart tonic, and it really cleanses the blood. Guduchi is known as a tonic for pitta, and pitta usually manifests with those fiery, heated emotions of anger, hatred, jealously. If you want to find that calm, Guduchi has an anti-inflammatory nature to it. It is really calming and soothing, and it's known as a rejuvenative—it helps rejuvenate the system. It helps support the nervous system, the effects of stress. Often when we feel that sense of stress, our immune system goes down, our nervous system goes down and then we tend to get sick. Guduchi really helps support those things. It is also a blood cleanser, so it helps remove all those toxic things that are coming out.

4. **Brahmi** is known for its balancing effect on the consciousness and in Ayurveda, the heart is known as the seed of consciousness. And so really, it is a matter of looking back, inward and finding that sense of inner peace and inner stability. Brahmi helps to bring that inner focus back and helps bring a calmness to the external focus that is really causing all of the nervous emotions—the unsettled emotions.

RECOMMENDED PRODUCTS FOR HEART HEALTH

- Heart Formula, Banyan Botanicals
- Ashwagandha, Banyan Botanicals
- Triphala, Banyan Botanicals
- Vata Massage Oil or Sesame Oil , Banyan Botanicals
- Deep Love Herbal Extract, Ayurvedic Institute, Dr. Vasant Lad

For more information on Ayurveda and Banyan Botanicals, check out heartbreakyoga.com

CHAPTER 11

Making Space

"My beloved child, break your heart no longer. Each time you judge yourself, you break your own heart. You stop feeding on the love which is the wellspring of your vitality. The time has come. Your time. To celebrate. And to see the goodness that you are . . . do not fight the dark. Just turn on the light. Let go, and breathe into the goodness you are."

—Swami Kripalvanandji (Bapuji)

LETTING GO IN THE MENTAL SPACE

Phase 1

IMAGINE YOU ARE AT THE BARNEY'S SAMPLE SALE (Macy's on Black Friday, H&M on any given weekend circa 5 p.m.). As you sort through the racks, dodging elbows with razor focus, you close in on The Prada bag you have been pining over. It's there, at the sample sale, how could this be?! It's behind glass with the new seasonals at Bloomies. There must be some amazing mistake. When you get to the register, the cashier reveals it is 70% off the already discounted rate. You shriek with excitement. You have scored!

You leave the store victorious, swinging the prized item onto your shoulder. However, it is heavy. It hurts. There seems to be something dense within. A look inside reveals that your brand new hobo bag is filled with the limitations of your last relationship: the time you bought a paycheck's worth of custom lingerie on La Cienega, and he wasn't "in the mood"; the Friday night you sat at home awaiting his call, only to discover his ex-girlfriend checking him in at a concert on Facebook.

Those old hurts are now oozing into the interior, staining this brand new beautiful bag!

How will you transfer the contents of your purse (including your hopes, dreams and yearnings) into this NEW bag, if all it's already filled with is all that OLD garbage? We need to clean it out—and how do we do that is by "Letting Go."

This lesson is brought to us entirely by the Godmother of Metaphysical Healing, Ms. Louise L. Hay, whose best-selling book *You Can Heal Your Life* has altered the course of millions of lives. She taught me one of the most important sentences I've learned to date: "I am willing to let go . . ."

Now you try. Say aloud, "I am willing to let go . . ."

Anything happen?

Feel a slight relief?

Okay, try again, aloud, "I am willing to let go . . . "

And again, "I am willing to let go . . ."

Aaaand again, "I am willing to let go . . ."

I invite you to continue saying this until you feel, hear or see a shift. It may be subtle at first, what feels like the loosening of a knot in your stomach, or a little more room around your temples. Hopefully, in time your shoulders will soften and your heart will open. Slow and steady wins this race too.

You might say something like, *"I am willing to let go of the time I bought a paycheck's worth of custom lingerie on La Cienega, and he didn't notice."*

"I am willing to let go of how much that hurt me, even if I didn't show it at the time."

"I am willing to let go of how embarrassed I was, when Diane asked

me how the striptease went, and I had to make up some silly reason why I didn't do it."

"I am willing to let go of my anger at the salesgirl for not letting me return any of the items, when I was already mortified (custom items, especially underwear, can't be returned. Duh)."

"I am willing to let go of any feelings of insecurity I now feel about sex or sensuality."

"I am willing to let go of how low that made me feel."

"I am willing to love myself for trying something new."

"I am willing to laugh at how awful that situation was."

"I am willing to call Diane and tell her the truth."

"I am willing to buy a new matching set of scandalous sentiments and wear them under my regular work clothes—HA!"

"I am willing to believe I can be beautiful and sexual just for me."

Try this for a week or so and see if that Prada bag gets lighter.

Phase 2

This is not for the meek of heart. Please do NOT skip right to this Phase.

Saturday Morning, 10:30 a.m. Coffee brews.

Heather and Amy sit at kitchen table.

Heather: This is either totally going to shock you, or you have already seen it 30 times today.

Reveal: TS's Facebook Page

In these modern times, the Facebook Stalk is the physical equivalent of driving past his house, stopping by his work or calling his friends— you know, just to check in, see what's up . . . *so, is he seeing that floozy or what?!?!?*

I dare you to limit your cyber drive-bys to once a day during business hours only. After a week of that, why not wean yourself to just one cyber-stalk a week?

You will be resetting the mental pattern and letting go of this masochistic behavior. Admit that every time you look at his page and see him engaged in an activity that does not involve you, it is a little bit like slashing your own wrist with kids' safety scissors. Yeah, it's not going to kill you, but it would be a lot more attractive to don a tennis bracelet without the scarring.

"I am willing to let go of looking at his Facebook Page."

See how that feels, and then when you feel REALLY daring, Un-friend him. You'll be amazed at how light That Prada bag suddenly feels.

Phase 3

What are some other things you may be willing to let go of? My first list went something like this:

I am willing to let go of sugar.

I am willing to let go of exercise excuses.

I am willing to turn my Blackberry off for one hour a day.

I am willing to let go of tardiness.

Your turn:

I am willing to let go of _____

_____

I am willing to let go of _____

_____

I am willing to let go of _____

_____

That Prada bag is lookin' good, girl!

LETTING GO IN THE PHYSICAL SPACE

Phase 1

Please tidy up the worn out, cried into copy of *The Notebook* and toss
the empty cartons of Ben and Jerry's.

Next: get those gross jammies into the wash, girl. Are you dressing
for bed like you have a lover, or like you are baiting the producers of
What Not to Wear for the $5,000 in free clothes? BE HONEST! Then get
rid of The Granny Panties. My publicist friend Lee Runchey's motto is
"You Get What You Get Ready For." Are you getting ready for Friday
Night with a hot new guy, or Ben, Jerry, Carrie and Big? BE HONEST!

Phase 2

This might hurt a little, so rip it like a Band-Aid—the quicker the better. Get his baseball socks, Bukowski book, Beta Band CD and blue
toothbrush into a box and into your closet ASAP. Yes, The Giants hoodie
that smells like him and the Bruce Springsteen DVD gotta go too. Mark
the date on the box. Promise that one year from today you will either
give these items back to the boy, to the garbage men or to Goodwill. As
we say in Sanskrit, "Swaha." Translation: "Into the fire," "Oh Well." In
other words, "To The Left!"

LETTING GO IN THE ENERGETIC SPACE

The Long Island Medium may not have the same style as you, but
when it comes to saging, sister knows her stuff. Referred to as a pri-
mordial ritual, the Native Americans have utilized sage smudging since
the beginning of their history. The technique is said to combine the
earthly world with that of the heavens, burning off heavy, dark, or negative energies, spirits and vibes. The yogis go-to for anything that feels
funky.

The Modern Day Version:

1. Purchase a bundle of sage at your local farmers market, health food store, or head shop.

2. Prep a glass of water, bowl and lighter or matches.

3. Hold the sage over your bowl

4. Set your sankalpa (your intention for this ritual).

5. Light it like incense. (When it catches fire, blow on it until only embers are glowing.)

6. Walk around the room circulating the stick. Don't forget the corners!

7. Personally, I like to thank all the energies for being with me, and politely ask those that no longer serve my highest good (some people call it bad, negative, static energies or entities) to move it on down the road.

8. As the smoke smolders and escapes out the window, maybe you want to picture your unhappy memories, or "stuck" scenarios escaping as well?

9. It's nice to say a little prayer in each room, resetting your sankalpa.

10. Give yourself a "sage shower." Cup your hands to catch the smoke and wash your body and face with it. As you do so, you may want to picture any unwanted or no longer needed energy or idea being carried off of you, on the smoke, out the window, into the ethos. If you take your own power back, that stuff can't hurt you anymore. *You are stronger than you think.*

11. Extinguish the flame in the way you best see fit. My dad the fireman will be infuriated I even put something so dangerous in print. He would want me to tell you to put it in the water. Do what you know is best for you.

12. But please double and triple-check to be sure the flame is out. Thanks!

LETTING GO IN THE PHYSIOLOGICAL SPACE

In yoga, it is widely accepted that the body is like tape recorder. The cells within our bodies, the ones that make up the tissues, organs and muscle, hold on to every experience on the cellular level. Much like how a song can transport you to a moment in time; the way a wheatgrass shot tastes; like getting kicked in the face in soccer; or how the smell of Nag Champa can bring you right back to the Freshmen dorms, so too can stretching, breathing and bringing energy (prana, life force) into long dormant parts of the body activate the cells, triggering a memory or emotion.

Back when I was a busy and important type, blackberry on vibrate tucked under my yoga mat, just trying out this yoga stuff (solely for the physical benefits of course), I begrudgingly experienced one of these emotional releases. This was back when I didn't believe in emotions, or their effects on the body. I had to run back to the office after class to grab the latest draft of the script. The producer and director needed my notes by morning. Who had time to care about things?

The room at YogaWorks was filled wall to wall while Travis Eliot (yoga teacher, kirtan wallah and friend to all) played the harmonium and chanted. Sara led us into an extended pigeon pose. The collective sigh of heavy exhales filled the sweaty, sagey, smoky room, with an energy all its own. I felt what I now understand to be an emotional release. Something long held within my hip (where we women carry a lot of our "Old Stuff"). I knew in an instant what it was. Something hurtful I had tucked away into the "I'll deal with this later" to-do pile in my mind. Well, poof! There it came out like a cloud of smoke, into the sky. My hip felt freer, lighter, more flexible. A few easy tears streamed down my face and then it was gone.

Typing with my thumbs, I ignored Sara's interrogation. I was very busy and important, after all. I didn't have time to talk about this. But, as always, Sara busted me. (Fist shake.)

Sara: *Ame, the class was very emotional tonight, wasn't it?*

Amy: Yeah, it was great, I love Travis. So do you want to grab a salad at Whole Foods quick? I have to get back to the office.

Sara: *Ame, did anything happen in class?*

Amy: Yeah, that good-looking guy from the co-op was checking you out the whole time. Do you think he is an unemployed actor and hangs there all day for handouts, or do you think he's like a Silicon Valley gagillion-aire that doesn't have to work and that's why he hangs there all day?

Sara: *Ame?*

Amy: Ugh. All right, yes, I felt a pop in my hip and then it was so weird I just started crying a little. I never cry. Well, I mean, I cry at funerals and of course, at the end of *Ghost* and *Goonies,* but I'm not one of those ridiculous, weepy, cry-y people.

Sara: (laughs) *You mean like me?*

Amy: Uh, yeaaah.

The usual yogis congregated with a round of "Congratulations," "That's Great," "Oh how wonderful," "Now do you get it?" It felt like a cross between the end of *Rosemary's Baby* (they're all crazy, I'm the only sane one) and the curiosity spawned from The Central Park scene in *Hair* ("Isn't this great?" "Aren't emotions wonderful?" "It's all in Technicolor?" "Hare Krishna!")

Amy: I've gotta get back to work. 'Bye guys!'

The Chorus: Namasté! Pranams! Congratulations, sweet Amy! Hare Krishna!

Yikes. What have I gotten myself into?

But a funny thing happened as I kept showing up on the mat and kept detoxifying my body of all the mental, emotional and chemical build up, I too started to think "Isn't this great?" "Aren't emotions won-derful?" "It's all in Technicolor." "Hare Krishna!"

Our emotions get trapped into the toxins in our bodies, which is believed to be a big cause of dis-ease. An acidic body is far more susceptible to illness—even mental illnesses, like depression. When we detoxify the system, we bring to it more energy, more vibrancy; we are able to make decisions from a place of clarity. All crucial elements in surviving a heartbreak.

In present day my friend, Naturopathic Doctor, and the founder/director of EcoHealth & Wellness of Charleston, South Carolina, Dr. Tiffany Jackson explains:

> Stress from a break up or unhealthy relationship causes the body to release certain chemicals that, if allowed to build up, are toxins in themselves. They disrupt the body's delicate biochemical balance. Research shows that a mental attitude has a huge effect in the outcome of treatments of various diseases. In Chinese medicine, the emotion of anger affects your liver function, worry will upset your digestive system, fear disturbs your kidney function, and grief damages the lungs.
>
> When you worry or are overly stressed out during a relationship, your adrenal glands over-secrete the stress hormones such as cortisol, which suppresses the immune system and upsets the nervous system.
>
> Stress from a heartbreak prevents liver detoxification. This is why I recommend doing a full-body Heartbreak Yoga 14-Day Detox.
>
> When you hear the word "detox," all kinds of things come to mind: juice fasts, colonics, rehab centers. People do detox programs to rid their bodies of toxins, lose a little weight, perhaps look and feel better about the damage they've done to their bodies. Specific detoxifications are recommended when you eat too many French fries, drink too many martinis and do too many drugs. But how do you detoxify from unhealthy relationships? Is there a solution for people who have had one toxic relationship after another? How do you take the damage done from too many bad relationships to enable a fresh start? A full mind-body-spirit overhaul.
>
> Amy: We don't need to check into Canyon Ranch Spa to fully detox do we? What's the wham-bam-thank-you-ma'am of bye-bye-heartbreak detox?

Dr. Jackson: No, you don't have to leave your daily routine to do a detox. I recommend a 14-day program. Detox helps you get rid of the toxins in your body and gives you time to heal on a physical and emotional level. During this 14-day time period you finally get time to stop, take a deep breath, detox your body and mind to get your romantic bearings in check. THIS IS "YOU" TIME! It's not about men, it's not about pleasing anyone else—you purely focus on pleasing yourself and healing your body and mind from the inside out.

Step 1: Eat a Detox Diet. A diet high in fatty, sugary and processed food, alcohol and stimulants dulls the communication between your mind and body because it puts a strain on your elimination system. A detox diet of alkalizing and nutrient-rich foods makes the communication system more vibrant. You will feel more energized, alive and mentally clear to go on dates after you do the detox diet.

Step 2: Take Supplements to Support Liver Detoxification. (See 14-Day Heartbreak Yoga Detox below.)

Step 3: No Alcohol for 14 Days [THE MOST CHALLENGING STEP]. Recommended Drinks: Drink only water, coconut water, and green tea.

Benefits of Coconut Water: The water from coconuts has a great supply of electrolytes. An 8.5-ounce portion has 15 times more potassium than most sports drinks, and is one of the main electrolytes your body uses to replace and retain the fluids needed to operate at full capacity.

Benefits of Green Tea: Historically, green tea has been used to treat a variety of health conditions in both Chinese and Ayurvedic medicine. Its use in detoxification is due to green tea's high polyphenols content. Polyphenols are powerful antioxidants that neutralize destructive compounds in the body known as free radicals. Furthermore, green tea promotes fat burning and facilitates weight loss. It never hurts to drop a pound or two before jumping back into the dating scene.

I took Dr. Jackson's advice and totally detoxified my already clean-running bod. I felt so vibrant, I want to share it with the world—so Dr. Jackson and I created a 14-Day Heartbreak Yoga Detox just for you!

14-DAY HEARTBREAK YOGA DETOX

One Heartbreak Yoga Detox Kit Contains:

- 🐨 1 Heartbreak Yoga Detox Powder

- 🐨 1 Heartbreak Yoga Detox Vanilla Powder

- 🐨 1 Heartbreak Yoga Detox (90 capsules)

- 🐨 1 Heartbreak Yoga Plant Enzymes Digestive Formula (90 capsules)

- 🐨 1 14-Day Heartbreak Yoga Detox/Cleanse Patient Guide

- 🐨 1 Blender bottle

- 🐨 1 Reusable bag made from recyclable materials

The 14-Day Heartbreak Yoga Detox/Cleanse Program has been created to support the body's natural two-phase detoxification process in order to safely and effectively remove harmful toxins from the body, and emotions too!

For more info, check out heartbreakyoga.com

CHAPTER 12

Beyond the Break-up

"Release Me"

—Pearl Jam

Sue: Who's coming to the dinner party tonight?

Amy: The usuals. Harry and Sally, Brad and Janet, Harold and Maude, Brenda and Eddie. Oh shoot! Should we invite Brenda or Eddie, or do you think it's time they learned how to be in the same room together again?

Tibetan Buddhism is a tradition firmly rooted in the belief of reincarnation. Births and Re-births. Multiple lives until the soul finds completion in its karmas (actions) and releases or liberates itself from this cycle of birth-life-death-rebirth called "Samsara" and moves into "Nirvana," the ultimate freedom/bliss/fulfillment.

While you are "In Bardo," you are in transition, preparing to make your move for the next lifetime. We learn about this in *The Tibetan Book of the Dead,* a book entirely dedicated to the preparation of death and rebirth. There it states:

"Now when the bardo of dying dawns upon me, I will abandon all grasping, yearning and attachment, Enter undistracted into a clear awareness

of the teaching, And eject my consciousness into the space of unborn aware-
ness; As I leave this compound body of flesh and blood I will know it to
be a transitory illusion."

Varun Soni, USC's Dean of Religious Life, clarifies:

In that moment, the clear light of bliss will manifest itself. The "pure light
of bliss" is sort of the nature of your own consciousness. When you die, if
you are familiar with this clear light of bliss, you will understand it to be
an emanation of your own consciousness. There's something that is imper-
manent and interdependent; it's not something that has ever been in exis-
tence, so this light that people see after they die is really a manifestation
of their own consciousness. So from the Tibetan Buddhist tradition, if you
understand that at the time you die you will achieve nirvana, you won't
come back into samsara, the cycle of suffering, you will basically be released.

Heartbreak Yoga Translation: If you prepare yourself for the death of
Brenda from "*Brenda* and Eddie," you might be able to liberate yourself
from the cycle of suffering.

Do you remember *Brenda* before she was *Brenda* of *Brenda* and *Eddie?*
Did Brenda have interests that Eddie didn't? Did some of these interests, ideas and even friendships fade into the compromise of couple-
dom? While you are "In Bardo" and accidentally catch yourself beginning
sentences with the pronouns "We" and "He" instead of wondering who
you are, why not simply remember? Why not make a list of Brenda's
interests and unexplored curiosities? It could look something like this:

- Turn YOUR music up as loud as YOU want when you get home
  from work.

- Have a dance party. Clothing optional.

- Finish that Jerry Garcia Jigsaw Puzzle you started in the Freshmen
  dorms.

- Commit to guitar lessons once and for all.

- Learn French . . . get ready for a lovah!

- Take a weekend wine tasting workshop.

- Watch *Pretty Woman, An Officer and a Gentleman* and *Dirty Dancing* in one sitting. I dare you.

- Make a playdate for yourself with a friend you haven't spent quality time with in years

- Send out the thank-you notes, wedding/baby/birthday/holiday gifts that are cluttering the "To Send" pile in your mind.

- Make your best friend a mixtape.

- Take the pole-dancing lesson you've been flirting around for months. Just doooo it. Life is short. No one will find out.

- Read all the great classic love story tragedies: *Anna Karenina, The Scarlet Letter, Romeo and Juliet, The Seagull.*

- Sign Up For MeetUp.Com, GroupOn, or a dating website. Ya gotta get back on the horse at some point. Might as well be with a total stranger. That way when you say something dumb, snarf your soup, or are just blatantly bored, the collateral damage is light.

In NYC:

- The Open Center

- The Art of Living Center

- Julia Cameron's *The Artist Way* Workshop

- Why don't you finally go to The Met, The Guggenheim, The Museum of Natural History? The Opera? Broadway? Off-Broadway? A Cabaret in The Village? An Ashtanga Moon Party in Brooklyn? What about The Blue Note? The Apollo? Why not take a tour of The New York Stock Exchange, 30 Rock, The Hotel Chelsea where Sid and Nancy are said to haunt the hallways? Go to Pete's Tavern at 55 Irving Place and sit in the booth where O. Henry wrote the best love story of all times, *The Gift of The Magi.* Then read *The Gift of The Magi.*

In LA:

- Bhakti Yoga Shala

- The Art of Living Center

- Julia Cameron's *The Artist Way* Workshop

- Have you ever actually been to The LACMA? Runyon Canyon? The Chateau Marmont? The site of the first Academy Awards,? The Hotel Roosevelt? Did you ever "Take Fountain" as advised by Bette Davis? If you go to The Hotel Continental, you can meet Janis Joplin's lover, Vernon, who still holds a vigil for her. If you wander into Laurel Canyon by way of The Country Store you can see where much of our classic rock n' roll music was born. That's where Crosby, Stills, Nash and Young; Frank Zappa; Alice Cooper; The GTOs; The Mamas and The Papas; Jackson Browne; Joni Mitchell; Eric Clapton; The Eagles; members of The Doors; The Stones and even The Beach Boys lived in the 60s and 70s. Just down the hill is The Troubador, The Whiskey-A-Go-Go, The Viper Room, The Roxy—all immortalized in our 80s and 90s rags to riches stories in *Behind the Music*. Check out The Canals in Venice where Jim Morrison wrote "Love Street." If you find yourself on the Venice Beach Boardwalk and meet Harry Perry (still skating around since *Fletch* and *LA Story*), please tell him I sent you. Thanks.

In Between NYC and LA:

- Sign up for the local community college or YMCA mailer.

- Julia Cameron's *The Artists Way* Workshop.

- The Self-Realization Fellowship provides mailed lessons to accepted applicants. The lessons are simple ideas techniques and stories as told by the Indian Saint, Paramahansa Yogananda who came to the United States in the 1920s. "Master" as he is called by devotees, served as a spiritual advisor to Franklin Delano Roosevelt, among other movers and shakers of the day.

Want to dive deeper into the spiritual classics? During your detox, why don't you build a bookshelf that looks like this:

- *The Seven Spiritual Laws of Success*—Deepak Chopra

- *You Can Heal Your Life*—Louise L. Hay

- *The Artists Way*—Julia Cameron

- *A Course In Miracles*—Marianne Williamson

- *The Eight Human Talents*—Gurmukh

- *Autobiography of a Yogi*—Paramahansa Yogananda

- *Be Here Now*—Ram Dass

- *The Tibetan Book of The Dead*

- *The Bhagavad Gita*

- And lest we forget, *The Gift of the Magi*—O. Henry (required Heartbreak Yoga homework)

For more information on all, please check out heartbreakyoga.com

"Be as simple as you can be; you will be astonished to see how uncomplicated and happy your life can become."
—Paramahansa Yogananda

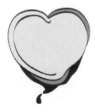

"Leave with dignity . . . Make your parting as sacred as your coming together. As the necessary means for new growth. You will not leave casually, but do not look back to do your loving in the sentimental past. Do it here and now with someone who may meet you in body, mind and spirit. Be prepared to have it all with them. Do not hold back based on past failures and fears, most of which are not your own."

—Mark Whitwell, *Yoga of Heart*

Ali: I left my knee socks & whistle at Biggie's the night of the Halloween Party. I'm going to pick them up tonight, what should I say if he asks about you?

Amy: Just your typical run of the mill "Worst mistake you ever made, buster" Laurel-from-Jerry-Maguire-like rant will do, thanks. Oh and if you see my dignity, would you mind grabbing it for me? I can't seem to find it here.

Ali: (laughs) I think I saw it in his upstairs bathtub.

Amy: (laughs) Goodbye.

Click.

DOs AND DON'Ts

Here are some tips on how to maintain your dignity throughout the break-up process, carefully procured from my amateur personal studies and observation of friends, colleagues, and summer camp bunkmates over the last 19 years:

DON'Ts

1. DON'T drink and dial. It will not be Robert Mondavi, Francis Ford Coppola or even Mr. Mad Dog's fault when you make ridiculous fan-

tastical statements on his voicemail. It won't be your friend Catherine's fault who ordered the second and third bottles of wine either. Only you are responsible for you. *You are stronger than you think.*

2. DON'T caffeinate and press send. It's my Rule #2. Not sure how I blew it on this one. Learn from my mistake kids, it's not worth it. Take a breather before sending "Hiiiiii Waaaaaayne" emails. You don't want to be the psycho-hose beast.

3. DON'T casually attempt to befriend his friends in order to keep tabs. Everyone from the Village Chief to the Counselors-in-Training will be on to you.

3.5. DON'T hook up with his best friend either. No one wins in the jealously game.

4. DON'T post self-taken sexy photos on Facebook. (Please see #s 3 & 3.5 above.)

DOs

1. DO surround yourself with people (and pets) who love you just as you are. If you have ever worked construction, sat on a barstool, or attended a Christian Church Service, you know that the Triangle, or the "Trinity" is the strongest structure. In Christianity it's "the Father, the Son and the Holy Ghost." In Buddhism, the triangle is called the Three Jewels: The Buddha, The Dharma and The Sangha. In its most crude translation, it means the Buddha Mind, the choice and commitment to the path of Buddhism; the Dharma means walking that path; and the Sangha means community to help you *stay on the path.*

The entire structure would crumble if one of them, say . . . the "Sangha" was missing. In addition to allowing love in, knowing that other people have endured the same, and feeling supported, your real friends are the ones who will wrestle your phone out of your tipsy-hand, and tell you not to press send. No man is an island. No woman will survive a tropical storm solo. Ask Amelia Earhart.

2. DO Shakti-fy! In Hinduism, the divine feminine creative life force energy is called "Shakti." Since the dawn of time, women have gathered together during their "moon cycle" to celebrate this sacred female power. In the midst of transition, my astrological fairy Godmother, Chani Nicholas, always pops up out of nowhere to remind me to be with my fellow females. She shares:

> *Sitting in circles is something that women have done since the beginning of time. We knew there was a cyclical connection between our bodies' cycles and the waxing and waning disk of the moon. Often women removed themselves from mundane life during their "moon time" to sit in circle with each other in order to receive the wisdom that is available to us at this time. Gathering together is powerful and necessary; we need to disengage from the world periodically in order to hear our inner voice."*

For more on Heartbreak Yoga community, check out heartbreakyoga .com

SATSANG (Community)

> *"If you want to work for world peace,
> go home and love your family."*
> —MOTHER THERESA

How many times have you been at dinner, and your view is of the crown of one or more of your friends/co-workers/children's heads? How many times have you been sitting in a room in a home and every single person's eyes are glued to an electronic devise—TV, iPhone, laptop, Gameboy? No one is talking. Everyone is click-click-clicking away.

I recently attended a family gathering, and such was the scene. I looked over at my 93-year-old grandmother and wondered where she thought evolution, technology and humanity would *choose* to take us. I pictured her and her sister, our Great Aunt Betty, playing piano together as young girls; boarding their shared bedroom during the depression; tending the family farm during the war; meeting their husbands at separate church dances the same year; sewing each other's wedding gowns; raising families a block away from each other; watching their five girls grow into women, all becoming mothers. The count is now 13 grandchildren and 14 great-grandchildren. I wonder if when they were playing dress-up as kids, daydreaming about the future, if they ever thought their great-grandbabies would be shushing their elders at the dinner table because they got to the next round of Angry Birds.

Is anyone else terrified of what we are letting technology do to us?

Did you know that nine months after a natural disaster, an extreme weather condition such as a blizzard, or a black out there is always a baby boom? It's true. Did you know they ran out of condoms in London during the Olympics? It's true. Did you know that babies of all species who don't receive affection die? It's true. Did you know that adult humans who don't receive affection die too? It's true. Dr. Peterson said so. Remember?

Voyeuristic techno-gossip gathered from the World Wide Web is not actual social interaction. Please go somewhere to be among real, three-dimensional people. Who knows—you might get lucky and meet your soul mate, or bump into Richard Branson giving out private islands. Crazier things have happened!

P.S. Call your mother. She's worried.

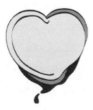

SEVA (Selfless Service)

> *"I do not know what your destiny will be,*
> *but one thing I do know:*
> *the ones among you who will be really happy*
> *are those who have sought*
> *and found a way to serve."*
> —ALBERT SCHWEITZER

In the Wavy Gravy film, *Saint Misbehavin'*, 60s icon Wavy Gravy speaks of a spiritual awakening:

> *"I realized that when you get to the very bottom of the human soul when the nit is slamming into the grit and you're sinking. You reach down to help someone who is sinking worse than you are, everybody gets high and you don't even need LSD to do that!"*

Wavy Gravy and his beautiful wife, Jahanara, have spent their lives helping people who are "Sinking worse." It began at Woodstock when Wavy Gravy was hired as head of security—the idea was no one would be able to run if they were laughing. Jahanara took on kitchen duty, preparing free food for the thousands of concertgoers who could not afford to feed themselves.

In 1978, Wavy Gravy, Jahanara, Dr. Larry Brilliant and his wife traveled to Nepal, where they were compelled to provide healthcare, nutrition and LAUGHTER to the impoverished of Kathmandu. They realized they could be of service in this way every day, and began the SEVA Foundation. Seva is the Sanskrit word for "Selfless Service." It is also known to mean "Compassion in action." Over the last 34 years, hundreds of friends have joined in this simple intention, among them are Ram Dass, The Grateful Dead, Joan Baez, David Crosby, Graham Nash, Ben Harper, Jackson Brown, and many, many devoted sevites.

SEVA's Sight Programs have restored vision to more than 3 million people in 12 countries by providing affordable cataract surgeries to people in some of the most remote places in the world.

SEVA's Native American Community Health Program has supported hundreds of grassroots wellness projects in native communities where health disparities disproportionately affect vulnerable, low-income people and are largely preventable.

When the nit is slamming against the grit, the dishes are mounting in the sink, the laundry is piling up in the hallway, the voicemail box is getting full and you just don't feel like any of it is worth anything anyway, why not be among those less fortunate?

Did you know one-third of the world doesn't have clean drinking water, and we flush after each time we use the bathroom? Did you know 50.7 million Americans are without health care? Did you know there are 67, 495 homeless in America? Did you know 12.8 million people are unemployed in the United States? There are 2.5 million orphans in Uganda due to the genocide? One million Sudanese have died as a result of The Darfur "Conflict"? Just some things to think about before sending out invites to the next pity party.

Every day is an opportunity to be "of service" to your fellow man, creature and even the earth. Here are some things you could do today: Walk dogs at the pound; read to the elderly; be a "Big Brother" or "Big Sister"; Meals on wheels; Mother's Kitchen; Hospice; teach yoga to prisoners, students and physically crippled; help high school students without parental support fill out college applications. If you are financially stable, why not buy an entire week's groceries for a single mom? If you are tolerant of, or even better, like children, why not babysit for friends so they can enjoy a date night? There are endless seva opportunities every day. Your soul will thank you! Your fellow human being will too!

GRATITUDE

> *"There are only two ways to live your life.*
> *One is as though nothing is a miracle.*
> *The other is as though everything is a miracle."*
>
> —ALBERT EINSTEIN

My Uncle Wally outlived his wife, five brothers, two sisters, endless friends and never had children. He spoke in reverie of "The Old Days," pulling coins from behind our ears, and telling silly jokes. When I would call to check in on him I'd ask, "How's it goin?" The response was always the same. "Welp, I woke up this morning, so it's a good day!".

He smoked, drank and read *Playboy* magazine until he joined his dearly departed. In all that time, Uncle Wally always found something to smile about. I continue to be enamored by his innate sense of appreciation.

The metaphysical translation of that outlook is called "Practicing Gratitude." In focusing our attention on what we are appreciative of, we are said to attract more of that thing (Love, money, *My So-Called Life* reruns). Regardless, of the material results, I'm often amazed at how this simple act can change my attitude while waiting on line at the post office, bank, or even DMV.

Mid mental-scream at the woman waiting in front of me for approximately ten minutes and eight seconds (but who's counting) and then did NOT have her mailing label/ deposit slip/ registration card filled out upon arrival at the window, I take a big deep breath in and on the exhale count my blessings. It goes something like this:

1. Thank you to Changing Lives Press for publishing this book.

2. Thank you to Francesca Minerva and Ellen Ratner for believing in me.

3. Thank you to Shari Johnson and Felicia Tomasko for the grammar lessons.

4. Thank you to my friends and family for *holding the space.*

5. Thanks for the tough love, life lessons and inspiration (you know who you are).

Why don't you try some?

6. Thank you to my mom for _____.

7. Thank you to my dad for _____.

8. Thank you to my dog/cat/gerbil for _____.

9. Thanks for the parking spot right in front of the door!

10. Thanks to the barista for always knowing my order.

11. Thanks to the copier for NOT getting jammed before the big meeting.

12. Thank you, body, for doing the breathing for me when I sleep at night.

13. Thank you to the God/Guru/Self for _____.

Got the hang of it? Okay, keep going . . .

14. Thank you to _____.

15. I am grateful for _____.

16. I really appreciated it when _____.

If you begin to love this practice as much as I do, you may want to start and end your day with it. My mom loves her 'Gratitude Journal." We each write down five things in the morning and five things at night, sharing at the year's end. Can you come up with 3,650 things to be thankful for? I bet you can! *You are luckier than you think.*

AFFIRMATIONS

"Keep your thoughts positive because your thoughts become your words. Keep your words positive because your words become your behavior. Keep your behavior positive because your behavior becomes your habits. Keep your habits positive because your habits become your values. Keep your values positive because your values become your destiny."

—Mahatma Gandhi

Did you ever have a friend who bought a Tesla Motors Sports Car, VW Bus, or Fiat? Suddenly, everywhere you go you see that Fiat: stop signs, the freeway, in your parking spot at El Porto. This is what is called a perception shift. Your brain now knows to register, "Hey look, a Fiat. It looks just like Vanessa's. Maybe it is Vanessa. HEY! VANESSA!!!"

It's as though you are playing Nintendo's Duck Hunt. You sit poised, waiting, at the ready for one of those animated ducks to come flying across the screen mocking your speed and agility. Quack-Quack. Quack-Quack. Quack-Quack. QUICK! What's the code to the extra lives in Contra? Up, up, down, down, left, right, left, right, b, a, b, a, select, start. If you are a video game kid of the 80s, you likely just accessed a file deep within the basement of your brain to pull up that data. You didn't know that filing cabinet was still down there did you?

Isn't the brain an extraordinary machine?

Like any machine, the brain runs best when taken care of; cleaned out, given the right power supply, and doing only the operations for which it was intended. Jim Jim Murphy has a brother-in-law that uses a chainsaw as a beer coaster. I mean, yeah, sure, I suppose it *does* protect the table from the ring caused by beer perspiration, but is that really the best use of that machine?

The same can be said of the three pounds and 100 billion neurons that make up the CPU responsible for transferring, filtering, and translating data in the body. Are you really using this high-tech server to the best of its ability? Have you learned how to use all the programs, or are you still running old scripts?

"He rejected me."

"What's wrong with me?"

"I'm unlovable."

"I'm ugly."

"I'm not good enough."

"I'm going to kill that bitch—how could she have stolen my man?"

Be honest with yourself. What is the default factory setting for your *computer?*

"I'm great. I'll be fine. I'm gonna make it."

Or

"Whyyyy meeee? Waaaah! I'll neeeevah looooove again!"

Your mental computer will continue to run the same scripts until you download the new software. Software like, "I'll be okay," "I'm beautiful," "Love is everywhere I turn," "There are plenty of fish in the sea."

There is a metaphysical practice called "affirmations" in which we affirm more of what we want:

"I am loving."

"I am lovable."

"I'm going to come out of this stronger than ever."

You may want to repeat to yourself:

"I am safe."

"I am happy."

"I am healthy."

"I am at ease."

Even dramatic ol' Scarlet O'Hara running around Tara, thinking she was the only person to be affected by the Civil War realized that strategy wasn't going to work. At the end of Act II, *Gone With The Wind,* she declared that she would nevaaaaah go hungry again. And guess what? She didn't.

SOME FUN HELPER-OUTERS

- thedailylove.com

- bighappyday.com

- behappy1001.com

- Notesfromtheuniverse.com (http://www.tut.com/)

"Mana eva manushyanam karanam bandha mokshayoho"
(As the mind, so the man; bondage or liberation
are in your own mind.)

—The Yoga Sutras of Patanjali

When I'm not checked into Heartbreak Hotel, my default setting world-view is that of a golden retriever pup about to score some bacon. *"Ooh, what's that over there? That looks like fun, let's do that!"* At first I found the practice of sitting still in meditation quite challenging. To be honest, I found it totally boring. Why sit still when there are SO many other cool things I could be doing? However, after experiencing the great sense of peace yoga asana provides, I thought I would give it an earnest, disciplined try. The people I knew who had a meditation practice were among the greatest, most grounded, fully clear and present. In addition, a lot of them were actually happy.

In fact, one of the happiest people I know is Maha Yoga's Steve Ross. Steve lived every teenage boy's dream of being a touring rock n' roll guitarist with huge name bands (the ones you have on vinyl, cassette, CD AND MP3—the ones you just keep buying and buying because they're that good). Steve loved his rock n' roll lifestyle, but began to love the simplicity of happiness without all the bells and whistles and tour buses more; the simplicity found in the quiet space of the present moment. It's from freeing his mind of all the limiting stories, ideas and cultural conditioning that he found:

"You are already happy. The reason you don't experience it is that it's covered up by layers of suppressed emotions and negative thoughts. Shift your attention and your inherent happiness flashes forth."

Sounds suspect, I know. Your brain might be bouncing around like a golden retriever pup that *didn't* get the bacon. *"But you said there would be bacon." "You said you would always love me." "I thought you would always be there." "What will I do now?"*

In yoga we call that the monkey mind. The monkey is always blindly, bumbling, grasping, and groping for another banana. Meditation helps to calm the monkey mind. It creates a discipline of your thoughts, so they're not swirling around getting sucked into the quicksand of "coulda-beens." Meditation anchors it into a place of stillness. Silence.

If we're going to learn meditation, I thought, best we learn the technique passed down from Buddha himself. The first human incarnate said to have attained enlightenment.

Meet David Nichtern. David is a senior teacher in the Shambhala Buddhist lineage of Chogyam Trungpa Rinpoche and Sakyong Mipham Rinpoche. He was one of the initial American students of Trungpa Rinpoche and studied closely with him soon after his arrival to the United States in 1970. David has been co-director of the LA Shambhala Center and Karme Choling Meditation Center in Vermont, as well as Director of Expansion for Shambhala Training International.

Without further ado, I give you David Nichtern . . . (And the crowd goes wild.)

CULTIVATING LOVING KINDNESS

by David Nichtern

The practice of cultivating loving kindness (maitri in Sanskrit and metta in Pali) is a Buddhist approach toward opening one's heart to others. It is very ancient, very simple, very direct and very effective.

The heart of the practice is generating four positive wishes for all beings:

May you be safe.

May you be happy.

May you be healthy.

May you be at ease.

We include beings we care for, those we don't care for, and those we don't care about. We even include ourselves!

Naturally it's easier to generate these positive wishes for our parents (in most cases), our children, our pets, our teachers, our friends. In that case, maitri or loving kindness flows unimpeded.

It is challenging to generate that kind of attitude toward people we are indifferent to and it is very challenging indeed to generate it toward people we don't like.

To prepare the ground for practicing maitri, it can be helpful to consider that the way in which we categorize other beings will change over time, sometimes very quickly, sometimes more slowly. Whatever we experience is subject to impermanence.

For example, an anonymous person we meet in the supermarket can become our lover and later on can become our wife and later on become our not so welcome (in some cases) ex-wife! We have gone through all three categories with one person.

Also, we can recognize that the way we look at people is very much related to causes and conditions. It is not absolute. If we are having a bad day, it is much easier to get irritated at somebody, maybe even somebody we fundamentally like. If we have had an abusive childhood, we can feel that the whole world is against us and we want to strike back. On a beautiful, sunny, spring day, sometimes everybody looks great and we are in love with everything and feeling groovy!

So causes and conditions set the stage for our attitudes toward the world and we can and do affect those causes and conditions. It is practical to train our minds further so that we are not governed by our negative habitual patterns.

And finally, it is worth noting and tuning into our most fundamental nature. What are we like when we are open, clear and fully present? What is our true nature? Do we really, really, actually wish others to suffer? Do we really, really wish to create the causes and conditions for our own suffering? What is wrong with cultivating openhearted and positive wishes for ourselves and others? Have we really become that cynical?

So practicing maitri is simple. Just take a comfortable seat in a quiet place and close your eyes. First think of somebody you love. Send them the four wishes. You can either repeat each for a time with that person in mind or just think about how those wishes might manifest and affect that situation. You can be creative about it.

Then move on successively to yourself, a "neutral person" (somebody you don't know well or already have strong feelings about), and then finally take the plunge and send the wishes to an "enemy." You may even notice that the choice of who the enemy is moves around and that's fine. As mentioned already, yesterday's enemy could be tomorrow's ally. Also, it's fine just to notice what comes up for you while you are trying to do this practice and simply allow space for that as well.

At the end, conclude by simply radiating out your loving kindness, your kind, sweet, loving open heart to all beings and send your good wishes to all of them (friends, oneself, neutrals, enemies, humans, animals, ghosts—anybody you can think of). Then simply dissolve the meditation and sit quietly for a moment or two.

This practice might feel too "touchy-feely" for some of us. At first I thought maybe it was too innocent, too sweet. But it is an ancient practice dating all the way back to the Buddha and it can be surprisingly powerful. It would be great if some of us who actually try it can write in and share their experience. Or, if you wanna be grouchy and just say something about it without actually trying it that's okay too!

Thanks, Dave Nichtern!

Think you are 2 keeeewl 4 skool and this loving kindness is for a bunch of tree huggers dancing around the desert barefoot? Well, yes, but also for some of our favorite urbanites.

If you were like me and spent the early 80s excited that video killed the radio star, wanting your MTV and fighting for your right to party, then you may remember a teeny little album, by a tiny little band called THE BEASTIE BOYS!!!

If you give the *Ill Communication* album a closer listen, not only will you be reminded how great Q-Tip and The Biz are, BUT . . . you will hear The Bodhisattva Vow, a promise written and rapped by Mike D, Ad-Rock, and that late, great Mahatma MCA. In the early 1990s, MCA took refuge in The Buddha. His loving kindness expanded exponentially as The Beastie Boys created the Milarepa Fund, an organization named after The Tibetan Saint Jetsun Milarepa who enlightened people through music.

Funny, I know three boys from Brooklyn who did the same.

Under the guidance of humanitarian and producer Erin Potts, the Milarepa Fund organized several concerts to promote awareness and raise capital for the Tibetan People.

From the original Milarepa.org website:

> *"Regardless of their philosophical, political, or spiritual beliefs, most people know that compassion and a responsibility towards others are essential for building a healthy society. The Tibetan people's struggle for freedom is the embodiment of a compassionate effort towards a strong community. In spite of the great political and spiritual upheaval caused by the Chinese invasion, the Tibetans have sustained their cultural celebration of non-violence and universal responsibility. The growing attention towards their plight shows the global desire to shift from physical, economic and military dominance to the use of compassion as a means to achieve change."*

These voices for change included The Red Hot Chili Peppers, The Smashing Pumpkins, Rage Against The Machine, Richie Havens, A Tribe

Called Quest, Pavement, Cibo Matto, Biz Markie, John Lee Hooker, Sonic Youth, Beck, Foo Fighters, Bjork, De La Soul, The Fugees, Buddy Guy, The Skatalites, Yoko Ono/Ima, No Doubt, Noel Gallagher, U2, Alanis Morissette, Patti Smith, The Jon Spencer Blues Explosion, Radiohead, Yungchen Lhamo, Ben Harper & The Innocent Criminals, Rancid, Pavement, Blur, Michael Stipe & Mike Mills, Taj Mahal and Phantom Blues Band, The Mighty Mighty Bosstones, Eddie Vedder & Mike McCready, KRS-ONE, Chuck D, Porno for Pyros, and Lee Perry featuring Mad Professor & the Robotiks Band, Sean Lennon, Mutabaruka, Money Mark, Dave Matthews Band, Nawang Khechog, Wyclef Jean, Herbie Hancock and the Headhunters, Buffalo Daughter, R.E.M., The Wallflowers, Blues Traveler, Live, Pearl Jam, Luscious Jackson, Run DMC, The Cult, Blondie, Tracy Chapman, The Roots, Handsome Boy Modeling School and Chaksam-pa.

Loving kindness is a lot kooler than you thought, huh?

Since May, Paul's Boutique, Phat Beats and The Brooklyn Skate Park have been missing someone. The Buddhist Temples of Nepal and The Bodhi Tree too. Sending a prayer that MCA graduated Samsara. (Xo)

Additional listening in this genre:

- Doug E. Fresh, "Pass the Buddha"

- Slick Rick, "Children's Story"

- Ice Cube, "Today Was a Good Day"

- 2Pac & Talent, "Changes"

- The Notorious B.I.G., "Juicy"

- MC Yogi, "Pilgrimage"

For additional meditation resources visit www.davidnichtern.com.

FORGIVENESS

"Always forgive your enemies; nothing annoys them so much."
—Oscar Wilde, Irish dramatist, novelist and poet (1854–1900)

Now when you are practicing your yoga and doing your morning meditation, you've let go, cleared the space and freshened your vibe. You look good, you feel good, you know you're gonna survive this, and then—boom! One of those crazy-ass psycho thoughts creeps in. You turn into Glen Close in *Fatal Attraction,* fantasizing about slitting his tires, maybe his new jogging partner's tires, or even your own. *"I don't want to go anywhere anyway. What's the point now that I'm not with him. Wah!"*

Instead of boiling up Bunny Stew, I invite you to clear out those pockets of your soul where the hurt is still stuck. We do this by practicing forgiveness. This can be quite challenging for some and easy as sweeping the dust bunnies out from under the couch for others.

There are plenty of people we can forgive. It can be the guy who never asked you on a second date, the job interview that went great but they hired the president of the company's niece, and yes, even (and especially) the bastard you had planned a life with, and was found sleeping with the next door neighbor. These are the carbon dioxide poisonings of karmic leaks . . . slow and silent, but ultimately deadly.

You may want to write a proverbial "never-meant-to-send" letter:

Dear _____,

   I forgive you for _____.

   Thank you for _____.

   I loved our times together/the opportunity to/ these traits about you _____.

   I was _____ to hear/find out/not hear from you. I am willing to forgive you because _____.

   I hope that you are willing to forgive me for _____.

   With love,

_____

It may not resonate as truth now, but I am proud of you for trying. It's brave to forgive. In doing so, you may deconstruct some of the ideas you had about "the whole thing." You may see that you played a part in the demise of your relationship—it's okay to forgive yourself for that too. We're all just doing the best we can. *You are stronger than you think.*

> *"Beyond our ideas of right-doing and wrong-doing, there is a field. I'll meet you there. When the soul lies down in that grass, the world is too full to talk about. Ideas, language, even the phrase 'each other' doesn't make sense anymore."*
>
> —RUMI

Sara: Knock, knock, it's me, Sara.

Amy: (Rolls eyes) Uh huuuh?

Sara: Ame, you always forgive and forget and then you get trampled by the same people and scenarios again and again. Remember what we were talking about recently when I said, "I don't understand—she keeps stabbing you in the back, and you keep handing her knives"?

Amy: Yeah, but I just can't believe she genuinely meant harm to me. She got confused. She's not a bad person.

Sara: Pretending that someone is good doesn't make it so. Being deluded and acting like someone didn't hurt you doesn't mean it didn't happen. It's true there is good in everyone, but not everyone is good for you. There's a modern Jewish proverb, "Forgive and remember." The holocaust was one of the most atrocious acts of terror in history. We don't forgive by forgetting. We forgive by learning from our mistakes so they don't happen again.

That Sara can be so annoying sometimes.
Especially when she's right.

MANTRA

"I forgot my mantra."
—JEFF GOLDBLUM IN *ANNIE HALL*

Zoë Kors is a cancer survivor. The 48-year-old single mom of a 16-year-old girl and a 5-year-old boy, Ms. Kors works as a branding and marketing consultant for your name boutique hotels that line the California Coast from Manhattan Beach all the way up to Malibu. In addition, she is the design director of *ORIGIN* magazine. Just in case that's not enough, at the urging of her clients, co-workers and kids, she relented and began a side business as a life coach to women who are juggling the same. Did I mention she's the first friend there with a tire-iron when you have a flat, or shows up unannounced with an organic, gluten-free casserole during a career crisis? Of course she is. So how does the unflappable Zoë Kors manage all this with a smile and style? She reveals:

> What has really become my strongest practice, what has sort of catapulted me to a whole new level is mantra. I chant every day. All day [laughs], honestly.
>
> When we talk about sankalpa, affirmations and things like that, real mantra, the way I'm speaking of it, is a series of Sanskrit sounds that resonate and activate different parts of the brain and really all the way down to the cellular level. Some are short. Some are long. Some are seed sounds. It is actually a vibratory sound. Some are names of Hindu Deities, or more conceptual, but it's a phrase that you repeat over and over again. It takes you out of your head. It's hard to describe what happens when you start to use mantra as a form of meditation. But, the best way I can describe it is, it takes you out of your head and into your heart.
>
> When I was designing the magazine recently, we were against deadline and I was working long, lonnnng hours. In the spirit of juggling many tasks at once, I would be able to just sit and chant mantras while I was working, which enabled me to be present in the moment and not get caught up in my head, in a state of overwhelm.

I find that in my life as a single mom of a teenager and a kinder-gartener, as I balance my needs, their needs, my practice and my career, and care of my parents who are in their 80s, it could be easy for me to be overwhelmed by everything and everybody that needs me. I find that when I chant, it keeps me in the moment.

Remember in the Indiana Jones movie *Temple of Doom* when Mola Ram pulls the heart out of a guy's chest and chants, "Om Namah Shivaya, Om Namah Shivaya, Kali Ma"? That's mantra. Those are prayers to Shiva and his consort Kali Ma, the male and female representatives of death and transformation in Hinduism. George Lucas knows what's up.

Remember in the beginning of the yoga practice when we learned the Guru Stotram? That's mantra. My Spidey sense tells me if you listen to George Harrison's first post-Beatle breakout single, the Phil Spector-pro-duced, "My Sweet Lord" you may hear something familiar. We have Mr. Harrison to thank for blending the spiritual with the material. First in the *Sergeant Pepper's Lonely Hearts Club Band* album, and then in his solo album *All Things Must Pass* (Ram Dass wrote the wave, George built the bridge).

If George can survive the breakup of The Beatles, we too can survive our breakup. Do you know how many teenage girls were at home cry-ing about the demise of the Fab Four? Probably way more than you'll have to inform when you change your relationship status. *You are stronger than you think.*

Harrison's re-birth record was heavily based on the following passage from The Bhagavad Gita:

> *"They are forever free who renounce all selfish desires*
> *and break away from the ego-cage of 'I,' 'me,' and 'mine'*
> *to be united with the Lord. This is the supreme state.*
> *Attain to this, and pass from death to immortality."*
> —BG 2:71–72

A mantra often recited at the close of yoga classes that speaks of the same theme is from the Upanishads. It is:

asato ma sadgamaya   (Lead me from the untruth to truth.)

tamaso ma jyotirgamaya   (From darkness to light.)

mrtyorma amrtam gamaya   (From death to immortality.)

—Brhadaranyaka Upanishad I.iii.28

My favorite mantra is: *Lokah Samastah Sukhino Bhavantu.* (May all Beings be happy, safe and free.)

Ya can't really argue with that.

Here are my Heartbreak Yoga modern mantra mix tapes. Pencil for rewinding not included:

TRANSFORMATION & LIBERATION

"Om/Invocation" • Steve Ross

"Mahaa Mrityunjaya (Om Triambakam)" • Ravi Shankar
    & George Harrison

"Jesus, Etc. (Live)" • Norah Jones

"My City of Ruins (Live from the Kennedy Center Honors)"
    Eddie Vedder

"Helpless (The Last Waltz)" • The Band ft. Neil Young

"I Shall Be Released" • Joe Cocker

"Om Mani Padme Hum (Long Version)" • Büdi Siebert

"Shiva Invocation" • Shantala

"Shanti (Peace Out)" • MC Yogi

"Wish You Were Here" • Vitamin String Quartet

"He Was a Friend of Mine" • Bob Dylan (The Bootleg Series)

"You're Missing" • Bruce Springsteen

"Sigh No More" • Mumford & Sons

"Shine a Light" • The Rolling Stones

"If I Ever Leave This World Alive (Live)" • Flogging Molly

"Everlasting Light" • The Black Keys

"Om Nashi Me" • Edward Sharpe & The Magnetic Zeros

"Shedding Skin (Beloved Friend Edit)" • MC Yogi

"Thank You (Live At Esplanade Arts) " • Chris Cornell

"Keep Me in Your Heart " • Warren Zevon

"Like Rain" • Jim Beckwith

"Beautiful Soul/Om Namah Shivaya" • David Newman

THE BREAK-UP BLUES

(Love, Denial, Anger, Bargaining, Depression and Acceptance)

"Dead Symphony No. 6: VIII. If I Had the World to Give" •
   Lee Johnson & Russian National Orchestra

"Sweet Thing (Live at Sin-e)" • Jeff Buckley

"Gopi Gita" • Karnamrita

"Unforgettable" • Nat "King" Cole

"Never Gonna Give You Up" • The Black Keys

"I Can't Hear You" • The Dead Weather

"Heartbreaker (Live)" • Nirvana

"Crazy Ex-Girlfriend" • Miranda Lambert

"Fuck You" • Cee Lo Green

"Song for the Dumped" • Ben Folds Five

"You Oughta Know" • Richard Cheese

"Emotional Rescue" • The Rolling Stones

"We Can Work It Out" • Stevie Wonder

"Don't Do It" • The Band

"Good Friday (Live at The Filmore)" • The Black Crowes

"Goodbye (Music from A Brokedown Melody)" • Eddie Vedder

"Mere Gurudev" • Krishna Das

"Last Goodbye (by Jeff Buckley)" • Vitamin String Quartet

"No Regrets" • Forest Sun

"No Hard Feelings" • Dinah Washington

ONLY LOVE CAN *HEAL* YOUR HEART

"Closing Time" • Tom Waits

"Walk Away" • Ben Harper

"Nobody Right, Nobody Wrong" • Michael Franti & Spearhead

"Time to Move On" • Tom Petty

"Sleeping Soul (Jiv Jago)" • Gaura Vani & As Kindred Spirits

"Karuna Sagari Ma" • CC White

"Lanka Burning (Sita Ram)" • Jai Uttal

"Township Krishna" • Krishna Das

"Sita Ram" • MC Yogi

"I Got Love for You" • Michael Franti & Spearhead

"Give Love" • MC Yogi

"Bold As Love (Live from Hampton)" • Phish

"I Love You and Buddha Too" • Mason Jennings

"Thanks and Praise (feat. Jasper)" • G. Love

"My Baba (feat. Krishna Das)" • Trevor Hall

"Rainbow (feat. Jack Johnson)" • G. Love

"Soulshine" • Gov't Mule

"You Can Count On Me" • David Newman

"NKB Kids" • Carolyn Shapiro & Friends

GOTTA GET *UP* TO GET DOWN (DOG)

"Last Thoughts on Woody Guthrie (Live)" • Bob Dylan

"Gotta Serve Somebody" • Shirley Caesar

"Riki Tiki Tavi" • Donovan

"Ganesha Sharanam " • Jai Uttal

"Jai Ma " • Wah!

"Krishna Love (feat. Jai Uttal)" • MC Yogi

"My Sweet Lord (Live)" • Billy Preston

"Amen" • Otis Redding

"Jesus on The Main Line" • Krishna Das

"Raise Your Hand (Live)" • Clarence Clemons

If you drink the Kool-Aid as quickly as I did, you too might free-fall down the rabbit hole and land at the "live in concert" version:

Bhakti Fest—The Spiritual Woodstock of the Decade!

On August 15, 1969, Bhakti Fest creator Sridhar Silberfein brought Sri Swami Satchidananda to The Woodstock Music Festival in Bethel, New York. There the Swami led about 500,000 people in prayer. His invocation is as follows:

My Beloved Brothers and Sisters:

I am overwhelmed with joy to see the entire youth of America gathered here in the name of the fine art of music. In fact, through the music, we can work wonders. Music is a celestial sound and it is the sound that controls the whole universe, not atomic vibrations. Sound energy, sound power, is much, much greater than any other power in this world. And, one thing I would very much wish you all to remember is that with sound, we can make—and at the same time, break. Even in the war-field, to make the tender heart an animal, sound is used. Without that war band, that terrific sound, man will not become animal to kill his own brethren. So, that proves that you can break with sound, and if we care, we can make also.

So I am very happy to see that we are all here gathered to create some sounds—to find that peace and joy through the celestial music. And I am really very much honored for having been given this opportunity of opening this great, great music Festival. I should have come a little earlier to do that job, but as you all know, thousands of brothers and sisters are on the way and it's not that easy to reach here.

America leads the whole world in several ways. Very recently, when I was in the East, the grandson of Mahatma Gandhi met me and asked me what's happening in America. And I said, "America is becoming a whole. America is helping everybody in the material field, but the time has come for America to help the whole world with spirituality also."

And that's why from the length and breadth, we see people—thousands of people, yoga-minded, spiritual-minded. The whole of last month I was in Hawaii and I was on the West Coast and witnessed it again.

So, let all our actions, and all our arts, express Yoga. Through that sacred art of music, let us find peace that will pervade all over the globe. Often we hear groups of people shouting, "Fight for Peace." I still don't understand how they are going to fight and then find peace. Therefore, let us not fight for peace, but let us find peace within ourselves first.

And the future of the whole world is in your hands. You can make or break. But, you are really here to make the world and not to break it. I am seeing it. There is a dynamic manpower here. The hearts are meeting. Just yesterday I was in Princeton, at Stony Brook in a monastery, where about two hundred or three hundred Catholic monks and nuns met and they asked me to talk to them under the heading of "East and West—One Heart." Here, I really wonder whether I am in the East or West. If these pictures or the films are going to be shown in India, they would certainly never believe that this is taken in America. For here, the East has come into the West. And with all my heart, I wish a great, great success in this Music Festival to pave the way for many more festivals in many other parts of this country.

But the entire success is in your hands, not in the hands of a few organizers. Naturally, they have come forward to do some job. I have met them. I admire them. But still, in your hands, the success lies. The entire world is going to watch this. The entire world is going to know that what the American youth can do to the humanity. So, every one of you should be responsible for the success of this Festival.

And, before I conclude my talk, I would like you all to join me and our group here in repeating a very simple chant. As I was reminding you of the sound power, there are certain mystical sounds which the Sanskrit terminology says are the bijakshara, or the "seed words." We are going to use three seed words, or the mystic words, to formulate the chants. And if you all join wholeheartedly, after the chant we are going to have at least one whole minute of absolute silence. Not even the cameras will click at that time. And in that silent period, that one minute of silence, you are going to feel the great, great power of that sound and the wonderful peace that it can bring in you and into the whole world. Let us have a sample of that now. The words will be: "Hari" is one word. "Om" is another word. The first chant will have these two words, "Hari Om Hari Om, Hari Hari Hari Om." The second line will be "Hari Om, Hari Om, Hari Hari Om."

There will be another chant afterwards: just one word, "Ram." We'll be repeating: "Rama Rama Rama Rama Rama Rama Rama Ram." It's a sample. It's very easy to follow with everybody and we'll have a gentle clapping also. So, now we'll begin in a slow rhythm and gradually build it up. Now I will request all of my friends to join me. We will repeat the line once, then allow you to follow. [The entire festival then chanted the "Hari Om" chant together.]

Thank you all very much. And once again, let me express my sincere wish and prayers for the success and peace of this celebration. Thank you.

Forty-plus years later a similar style crowd (and some of the originals) join together and chant the same names. For more info check out: www.bhaktifest.com and heartbreakyoga.com

Hari Om!

"A little louder, with your heart."

—HK Madhava Prabhu Ji

Did you ever wonder what those beaded necklace, bracelet-y things that yogis wrap themselves in are all about? My good friend (and former roommate) Vanessa Harris, creator of One-O-Eight Malas, is going to tell us:

Amy: Vaness, why did you drop everything to start making malas?

Vanessa: On a recent pilgrimage to India, His Holiness Indradyumna Swami shared the essence of Mala Beads. "Mala beads are our umbilical cords to the Divine—they are direct connection To God." Mala beads, known as the original rosary bead, are used in many prominent religious traditions as an aid to facilitate one's practice of meditation, of having our mind elevated and fixated on the Divine. It is believed that all sense is given to us as various means of experiencing, or spirit. Thus, by holding a mala, we are able to experience through the sense of touch. By both touching the mala and repeating in chanting mantras, a practice known as "japa yoga," we cleanse our hearts and minds of mundane, material thoughts and move a little closer to our more natural and Divine essence.

I sat on my balcony at the Ashram in Mumbai and realized this ancient tradition is just what we need in this rapidly evolving day and age. By submerging into the abyss of Japa Meditation and chanting the holy name on Malas, we do not get stuck in our own heads, but get out. Our mentality and thought patterns change. We go back to our simple childlike nature. We remember God. All self-defeating thoughts and anxieties and lists of to-do and to-don'ts that our over-stimulated culture seems to instill naturally just vanish. We return to the heart.

Amy: 108 is obvs the lucky number of Hinduism, due to the Muktiko-panishad Upanishads, but why are there 108, 54 or 27 beads in a mala?

Vanessa: There are usually 108 plus the Guru Bead. The auspicious-ness and sacredness of the number 108 is prevalent in many religions. In Hinduism, deities are known to have 108 names. In Buddhism, it is believed that there are 108 defilements, thus each bead represent-ing one of the 108 earthly temptations a person must overcome to achieve nirvana. It is also reflected in the 12 zodiac signs and the 9 planets.

Amy: Which in numerology breaks down to three, correct?

Vanessa: Correct.

Amy: Why did I hear you chanting like a songbird every time you made a mala?

Vanessa: The best way I can explain this is through the understand-ing of prasadam. Prasadam is food offered first to God before eating.

People chant while cooking prasadam. The food is filled with love, consciousness and intention of those making the food. Lots of times we get layered by others' consciousness without even knowing it. Look at the food—it's all about the cook. Say he is wildly enraged about something—the food may come out richer or spicier, which affects those who eat it. The recipients carry that karma with them. It's as simple as they could get a stomachache and have a bad day. It is important for the cook to have good, perhaps even God consciousness. That is why cooks chant while making prasadam.

Making malas is like making prasadam. Sure, people don't eat malas, but we definitely carry the vibration of the beads, the clothes we wear, etcetera. That is why it's important to know that your clothes, jewelry and so forth are being made in good consciousness, not slave labor. This is why I chant and make a ritual out of making malas, and offer them to God like we do with our food: to clear the karma of the beads and the recipients. The minute I sit down to make malas, I light incense to clear the space, sit in front of my altar, chant to and think only of God, as that is what malas are supposed to do anyway; remind us of God. I don't let a stressful relation or bad workday go into the malas, because that will go with them. They are tools for love, so they must be made with love. Consciousness is everything.

Amy: Thanks, Ma. Do you want this *Cosmo* mag when I'm done with it?

Vanessa: Yes. Here's the copy of the *Rig Veda* you wanted to borrow.

Amy: Radhe!

Vanessa: Shyam!

MALA MAKE UP

Malas are usually made from:

Rudraksha—"Rudra" is a synonym for Shiva, the God of Transformation, and "aksha" means "eye." Therefore, rudraksha is known as "The Eye of Shiva." Rudraksha trees are said to grow from the tears of Shiva, a powerful catalyst for change.

Tulsi—"The Incomparable One"; Tulsi has been worshipped for thousands of years as a physical manifestation and embodiment of Mother Earth.

Sandalwood—A peaceful, soothing wood, whose fragrance is known to promote tranquility, clear thinking and positive vibrations.

Crystal—Contains healing properties to the body, mind and psychic space. It amplifies healing and positive vibrations, dispelling negative energy and confusion.

Pearl—Known to contain strong healing powers for the body while promoting purity, honesty, peace and patience.

Malas can be purchased from your local yoga studio, health food store, temple, ashram, event or from the Heartbreak Yoga Website.

Once selected, choose a mantra you will use during this practice. It can be the Holy Names bestowed upon you by a Guru or teacher; you can choose a mantra for yourself (I cannot recommend one for you); or simply use an affirmation you feel strongly about, as "I am at peace," or "I am at ease."

HOW TO USE A MALA

1. Hold the mala in your hand.

2. Close your eyes

3. Feel the guru bead in your hand. Move your fingers to the next bead. Hold the bead between your thumb and preferred finger.

4. Beginning with that bead, chant your mantra or recite your affirmation.

5. Allow your thumb to pull your mala to the next bead. Recite your mantra or affirmation. (If you keep the mala draped over your hand, it will caress a meridian point, helping to achieve the desired "At Peace" effect).

6. Continue this practice until you reach the Guru Bead

   • You may want to say a special prayer once you reach the Guru Bead.

   • You can continue by going BACK around the mala from whence you came, or simply end the practice there.

The intention is to direct your attention away from chaos and self-defeating thoughts and into a state of directed, calm, focus. Japa (the use of a mala) combines mantra/affirmation with acupressure, union with sacred materials (rudraksha, tulsi, sandalwood, crystal or pearl) and of course meditation. Fashion AND Function—it's like the divine version of a Diane Von Furstenberg.

Mahatma Gandhi perpetually practiced japa meditation. His mantra was the name of his God. While Gandhi passed the bar exam, protested the British imposed salt tax, calmed the carnage between Muslims, Hindus, and Sikhs, while he was imprisoned for political protest and even as he lay dying, Gandhi repeated: "Ram, Ram . . ."

CHAPTER 13

And More Practice

"Do your practice and all is coming."
—Sri K. Pattabhi Jois

Nineteenth-Century Muslim-Hindu Saint Sri Sai Baba of Shirdi once said of spiritual practice:

"Beginning with simple repetition, gradually but inevitably, the Divine power which is hidden in it, is disclosed and takes on the character of a ceaseless uplifting of the heart."

GRADUALLY BUT INEVITABLY . . .

I learned this from Krishna Das.

Krishna Das is a well-loved, highly respected teacher whose workshops and retreats consist of dharma (spiritual) talk and "Kirtan" a call and response-style singing, using the sacred syllables and seed sounds of mantra. The whole scene is a lot like the old Gospel Churches I would visit in Harlem. "Can I Get An Amen?" "Amen!" "I said, can I get an AMEN?"

"Aaaaamennnnnnnnn!"

A Rick Rubin-produced, Grammy nominated, World Music Chart topper, KD is often referred to as "The Mick Jagger of Kirtan," but I liken him more to Ray Charles. Smooth, soulful and only has eyes for what's going on inside. I'm waiting for the hit single, "Maharaj-ii on My Mind."

In my ten-plus years in the film industry, not once did I stagger, shy or get star struck. Be it a Martin Scorsese, Sydney Pollack, or *Sex and The City* set, I was Miss Cool Cucumber. One "Om" from Krishna Das (KD), and I go more Beatlemania than a teenybopper outside Justin Bieber's Bentley. "I have all your albums!" "I loved your book!" "Will you sign my cartals?!" The harder I try to "Stay Calm and Chant On," the more embarrassing the things are that come out of my mouth. I make that awkward *Dirty Dancing* moment in which Baby tells Johnny she carried a watermelon look like the cooooolest thing anyone has ever said. Every time I talk to KD, I am carrying a *kirtan wallah watermelon*.

During his recent residency in LA, KD repeatedly reiterated the importance of repetition:

> **Gradually but inevitably.** Gradually but inevitably. I love that phrase
> . . . Let me start where I am. I'm here, I know I'm here. Now what's
> in here? Who is here? That's what I want to know. My belief is that
> what lives within me is that divine reality. All I have to do is uncover
> it. The path is a personal, individual quest for each of us. It is a jour-
> ney of spirit, not necessarily having to do with organized religion.
> When we can live in spirit, meaning that which lives inside of us
> already, we will see everywhere.

Gradually but inevitably if we keep showing up, keep getting on the mat, keep doing the practice, something will shift, something will move. We can begin to breathe again, believe that we might make it another day, believe . . . as Krishna Das's Guru, Maharaj-ji (Sri Neem Karoli Baba) would say . . .

"Sab thik hojaega" "Everything will be all right."

AND NOW A WORD FROM THE EXPERTS . . .

Lauren Eckstrom—Yoga Teacher, Santa Monica, CA
"In the Bhagavad Gita, Krishna gently tells Arjuna, 'You can't be anyone you want to be because you have to be yourself.' **Gradually but inevitably** our yoga practice unfolds in the same way. As we journey deeper into the space of mind, body, breath and soul unification we discover, gradually but inevitably, an art of practice that is uniquely our own."

Clayton Campbell—Kirtan Cajon Drummer, Los Angeles, CA
"Kirtan opens me up to my truest self. Even in the fire or the toughest days, the chants bring me home. Just like KD sez, **'gradually, but inevitably.'** We all come back to our true home within. Ya just gotta keep keepin' on!"

Pascal LaPoint—Kirtan Artist, Minneapolis, MN
"Whenever I get impatient on my path, KD's words come to mind: **'gradually, but inevitably'**—and my heart relaxes in the knowledge that there is no need for haste. All love!"

Sarah Ezrin—Yoga Works/ Power Yoga/ Equinox Yoga Teacher, Los Angeles, CA
"If you show up every day on your mat, **gradually, but inevitably**, your true self will be revealed."

Joanne Cohen—Sacred Goddess, Los Angeles, CA
"Sometimes when my heart is closed off and protected and I am longing for it to burst open, I think of how Krishna Das says **'Gradually but inevitably'** . . . and I relax into knowing that my heart is always returning to its natural state of oneness."

Mas Vidal—Dancing Shiva Yoga and Ayurveda, Hollywood, CA
"'Gradually' our life improves when we make the spiritual effort Now. '**But inevitably**' our smiles get bigger and our hearts open wider as we get closer to the One."

Neem Das—Kirtan Wallah, New York, NY
"Our true essence laughs at what the ego strives for. But it is that striving from the ego which catapults us for lifetimes, until a gentle wave of grace awakens us to a new reality. '**Gradually, but inevitably**,' as Krishna Das says, we finally 'get it.'"

Hanna Joanne Klausner—Marriage and Family Therapist, San Luis Obispo, CA
"I make things so hard for myself sometimes . . . then eventually I get tired of holding on to the way I think it should all be. Like KD says, '**Gradually but inevitably**' I once again remember to let go and flow . . . and often it all turns out better than I could have planned. Wooooot!"

Michael Stebbins—Teacher Bhakti Yoga Shala/Architect, Culver City, CA
"How does the spirit part find its way in? As Krishna Das states, '**Gradually but inevitably**.'"

Bianca Mora—Mora Management, Santa Monica, CA
"When my mind is racing and I find myself consumed with searching for answers, I remind myself, '**gradual but inevitable**,' all thanks to The Man, 'KD' Krishna Das."

Stephanie Lana Ramapriyan
"KD's quote, '**Gradually but inevitably**' reminds me that the dreams in our hearts and mind's eye will come to fruition with patience. It also reminds me to surrender from attachment of the outcome and not to give up on your dreams. Our

daily practices will **gradually** lead us toward the **inevitable** place of well-being. Chant, do yoga, meditate, take care of your health and persevere with action."

Ashley Wynn—Yoga teacher, Kirtan/Hug-Sharing Lover, Las Vegas, NV
"When I am stuck in my head, KD's words fill my heart and bring me back into that place of love . . . **Gradually but inevitably** . . . smiling all the way!!!"

Philippo Franchini—Bassist
"**Gradually** the sweet nectar of bhakti wears down the coarse rock of selfish, fearful resistance, and the idea of separate self **inevitably** melts into the blissful Union of Divine Love."

Dearbhla Kelly, M.A., Los Angeles, CA
"As I approach 40 and take stock of what I've learned, here's one thing: when you feel that deep pull from the depths, the one you're afraid of, the one you stay busy to resist, give in. Surrender. Immerse yourself in the blackness and discover this great secret: at the center is a seed of light. Its rays will shine on you, will slowly melt the hard core of whatever is crushing your soul. **Gradually, but inevitably,** your light will intensify until you emerge on the other side, the luminescence of your very being lighting the path all around you."

Rachel Weber—Archaeologist-turned-yoga-teacher, Starfish Yoga, Ana Maria Island, FL
"I was terrified before teaching my first yoga class. I wanted to throw up, but the students were counting on me, so I pulled it together and led them through a slow vinyasa flow. I was pouring sweat, as the nerves began to subside. By the end of class, I felt great . . . I am a yoga teacher! But before teaching my next class, the anxiety and fear returned, and again before the one after. I began to wonder if the nerves and nausea would always be a part of my teaching experience. **Gradually but inevitably**, I didn't have a moment of nausea today, and teaching yoga is total joy."

Alison Bryce—Project Analysis/Wellness Layers
"On the days that I wake up with little inspiration, energy or calm, I do a quick kneel at the foot of my bed and slowly repeat KD's words, '**gradually, but inevitably.**' These gentle words work in a profound way to instantly relax and restore me. I stand back up, a little taller than before, knowing that his words are truth—with patience and devotion, we're all headed Home."

Zat Baraka—Breathwork Teacher
"When I want to free myself from the need to look like a perfect LA urban Yogi, I just remember what Krishna Das told me, '**gradually but inevitably.**' "

Noah P Christensen—The Ultimate Yogi Program
"Things take time baybay. **Gradually, but inevitably.** Hello!! Don't you listen to Krishna Das?!"

Brenda Patoine—www. TheBhaktiBeat.com
"In the West we want everything fast, right? Fast food, fast trains, fast credit . . . It's the twitter mentality: give it to me in 140 characters or don't give it to me at all. So, when we start 'waking up'—maybe getting little glimpses of higher consciousness, of the oneness that unifies us all, of The Divine Light Within— we want that fast too. Instant Enlightenment? Sign me up! Chanting the names, they say, is one of the fastest ways to God-realization; I don't know about you, but that has a lot of appeal to me. But guess what? It ain't gonna happen overnight! You can be 'In the Bhav' for four glorious days at Bhakti Fest and you may feel like you've transcended straight into that sweet spot of blessed inner bliss and you ain't ever coming back . . . then you go home to a stack of bills and a pile of dirty underwear and reality slaps you in the face. Where's the bhav now? **Gradually but inevitably**, folks, just like the Chant Master says."

Sara Ivanhoe
"I was a hot mess. What was I forgetting? Keys? Check. Phone? Check.
Headset? Check. Does the dog have water? Do I have my water bottle?
Did I drink enough water today? Check. Check. Check. Hmmmm . . .
MY ANXIETY! WHERE WAS IT? I couldn't seem to find it anywhere and
didn't know how to leave the house without it. Just when I least expected it—
all that practice actually worked? Huh—I don't know what to do now.
'**Gradually but inevitably.**' Thanks, Big Red."

Ragani—Kirtan Artist, Milwaukee, WI
"Wait . . . what?! And all this time I thought Krishna Das had been saying,
'**Gradually but irreverently**' . . ."

Amy Beth Treciokas—Founder, YogaNow, Chicago, IL
"Once I asked Krishna Das if it was okay to combine a Krishna chant with a
Shiva chant. He touched me on the nose and said, 'There are no rules in love.'
And I realized that **gradually but inevitably** it all turns to love."

Michael H. Cohen—Dattatreya Kirtan Artist, Detroit, MI
"Pilgrims arriving for a blessing by the renowned Indian Saint Shirdi Sai
Baba were frequently asked for 2 rupees. These rupees represented each
aspect of his famous saying, 'Shraddha and Saburi' (practice and patience).
The deep truth hidden in Shirdi Baba's concise instruction is that by faithfully
engaging with an authentic spiritual practice (such as Kirtan) over a period
of time you will invariably see dramatic shifts in who you are being. Through
the practice of Kirtan you build deep connection with your body. Your mind
quiets and becomes receptive while your heart opens and extends. You begin
the journey through your heart to the Heart of the Divine . . . and beyond.
In this way, as Krishna Das is fond of saying, **gradually, but inevitably** you
are transformed."

Jeremy Frindel—Director, One Track Heart: The Story of Krishna Das
"Real, deep, change doesn't happen overnight. It comes over time, through
constant practice. 'Gradually, but inevitably.' With patience, perseverance, and
steady practice all will be revealed. Inevitably! At least that's what they say. "

Jim B. Gelcer—Kirtan Artist, Toronto, Canada
"Why do all the great sages, from Savanna to Pattabhi Jois to Neem Karoli
Baba and beyond, speak of the importance of daily practice? Whether it's asana,
meditation, chanting, or some other form of yogic practice, this seems to be a
universal teaching. I'm no sage, so I can't tell you. **Gradually but inevitably**,
though, I aim to find out."

Devadas—Kirtan Wallah, New York, NY
"I've heard my Guru liken spiritual growth to the budding of a flower; that
with the necessary conditions and patience we should have faith that the heart
will open and bloom like a rose, that **gradually but inevitably** we will become
who we are. While I believe this to be true, accepting this idea while navigating
a spiritual path in our day-to-day world is not always particularly easy. Life still
happens, the good and the bad. We make mistakes, we have bad days, and we
all have to deal with circumstances that are often beyond our control. And
while sadhana doesn't necessarily change those things, I've found, in my limited
experience, that it has shifted my perspective and the way I deal with life's ups
and downs, stutters and starts. To me, this is the real immediate grace of a
consistent practice, to be able to live with more ease, more acceptance, and
more empathy. And while the beauty of the rose's full blossom might be left
to our imaginations for now, this grace, this change in perspective, fuels my
faith in its inevitability."

Sruti Ram—Sri Kirtan
"When I think of Maharaji and KD and the shakti that Maharaji shares
with him; I would say that KD is fulfilling Maharaji's vision **gradually, but
inevitably**. Guru's grace is the most powerful energy a person could attain in
a lifetime, Ram Ram."

Julio C Andujar—DJ Lakshmi, San Diego, CA
"I remember my Yoga Teacher Jessica taking me to my first Krishna Das
Kirtan in Hawaii. I wasn't feeling very spiritual that day and the idea of going
to a sing-along sounded ridiculous to me at the time. I tried to hide in the
back, but my teacher skillfully placed me directly in front of KD's cushion,
center stage. I reluctantly awaited this ultra-holy Mila Repa character to
materialize in front of me and out comes this scruffy dude with a red plaid
flannel on. He looked and felt like everything I needed to see at that very
moment to simply pay attention. At first he seemed as disinterested as I was
when I arrived. All these people were clamoring over him and he was so
gracious, but kinda over it. He took his seat in front of me gave me a subtle
yet mischievous grin and then the magic began. As he chanted, spoke and
prayed with us . . . I softened, cried and released so freely. All the while
realizing he is the perfect mirror of love and spiritual perseverance for my tribe
and generation. He told us that chanting was 'medicine to heal our hungry
and broken heart' and that even if we didn't feel anything now '**gradually but
inevitably**' it would have an effect. He was and is so correct. Krishna Das
embodies the message of the Saints through his devotional practice, which
helps us know and understand the parts of ourselves we think no one else
could love. He truly is one of God's children who has bravely led millions
to the party in their hearts through grace, humility and honesty. Bravo.
JAI BHAGAVAN!"

Ishwari—Sri Kirtan, Woodstock, NY
"We perceive life as a journey that gets us from point A to point B. There is
a lot of anxiety about arriving at that imagined destination. But as KD says,
"**Gradually, but inevitably** . . . " only to realize there was nothing other than
Love we were after. I guess we all like traveling better than arriving. Maybe
we like to play hide and seek. Why? I don't know, but I imagine one day we
will grow tired of the games and just surrender.

Ambika Cooper—Kirtan Walli, Seeker/Mother
"That phrase '**gradually but inevitably**' turns my mind around completely—
in a good way. It remains one of my favorite stories from Krishna Das—about
the seeds that blow and then land on a roof, taking root slowly over time. I
love the promise of "**inevitably**." It gives me greater perspective and helps me
to take a step back from the quagmire of my thoughts. With that inevitability
in mind I can relax my grip a bit, and patience feels more possible (I am an
impatient type at best). The practice of chanting has become an anchor for
me; it is a refuge I can take each and every day. Much gratitude to KD for
bringing these practices and stories to us all."

Brenda McMorrow—Kirtan Wallah, Ontario, Canada
"To Be THAT, to rest in the place of Truth that is beyond words and beyond
concepts is '**Inevitable**' because it is What I Am! And even when I forget, I
can relax and know that the remembering is always possible. No need to rush
or get anywhere, it will unfold perfectly. All I need to do is open my heart
and be willing. Even be willing to forget! I love KD's words '**Gradually but
Inevitably**' because I am reminded to simply surrender into that which I
already am."

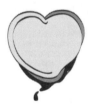

GRADUALLY, BUT INEVITABLY: MO THE YOGA DOG

A story by MC Yogi, as told to Amy Dewhurst

When I came to yoga, I was so numb, I was in so much pain, so much anger, so much hatred. Ya know all the things that happened to me when I was young. I felt angry at the world, and angry at myself and angry at God, and angry at everyone. It was through the practice of yoga that I was able to offload all that. I was able to stand up again. I was able to move.

That is one of the definitions of ecstatic. Static means to be stuck and 'ex' is like exodus, 'to leave,' 'to break out.' So yoga is the practice of breaking out of being stuck. Clearing the path so you can move again. It's like traffic opening up on the LA freeway; it's a miracle. That's what it was—it was like this miniature miracle I experienced. It was a small thing, but for me it was really big.

And Mo has the same story as me, man.

We rescued Mo from the East Bay. His real name is Mahatma Hanuman Shakti. When I first met Mo, I couldn't even approach him, he was so fearful of men. He was barking and so angry and upset. Scared—just like shaking and petrified and in this mode of protection. He would just bark at everything that moved; he was just a wreck. But I had this feeling when I first saw him—I felt like he was my old friend. I felt like I recognized him.

My dog is not like a pet. My dog is my friend.

Someone had found Mo in a parking lot. He had been abused by some people. When I met him, I just knew—it was the soul recognition. Same thing when I met Amanda [his beautiful, artist wife]. Like I knew right away that we were going to get married. In fact, I had a premonition before I met Amanda.

The closer I got to the day when I was going to meet her, I felt like she was getting closer and closer and closer. We met the first day of our yoga teacher training that was being taught by my teacher Larry Schultz, who used to teach for the Grateful Dead. He had one of the first big vinyasa yoga studios in San Francisco. He was a legend. So Amanda walked in and I just instantly recognized her and I knew I was going to marry her. But none of it made sense. Like from a rational place, nothing fit. The math didn't work out.

Same with Mo. I couldn't even pet him. I couldn't even get near him. Why would I want to take in this dog that doesn't even like me?

Life is like that sometimes. There will be people you just do not like at all that turn into your best friends.

I told Amanda I was getting this strong hit. I mean I was like in love with Mo, dude. I was dreaming about him and I couldn't stop thinking about him. So we decided to take him and at that time we had just opened the yoga studio. We would take Mo to yoga with us. He would plunk down right in front of the heater and he would just soak up all the heat—just lie there while everyone was doing yoga.

In the process of going to all those yoga classes, Mo healed himself, because he was around humans who were in a relaxed mode. All of them breathing, all focused on their inner work—class after class, week after week, year after year, '**gradually but inevitably**,' as our friend Krishna Das says, I watched him melt. That's why he's a yoga dog. And, he's a Pit Bull. There's a lot of baggage around Pit Bulls because of how human beings treat them.

Gradually but inevitably, whatever you give love to is going to thrive. Whatever you give love to is going to just grow and blossom and be successful.

So Mo came to every yoga class, sat in the corner, it was hot, people were chanting 'om,' doing their practice. He would lie in between, on people's feet in Savasana and he just gradually healed.

To me, it's this time-tested process; it's like the journey around the mountain. It's like the practice on the mat. It's when we sit on our cushions, it's like, when we do the work—it works. But you gotta just keep showing up. You gotta keep breathing, keep doing the mantra, whatever the practice is. You gotta just keep doing it. Don't stop.

"Get those children out of the muddy, muddy . . ."
—Folk Song "Rise and Shine"

It is said that it takes 40 days to break a habit or create a new one. Check out this list of new habits we've learned about. Then, for each day that you try one, add a heart to your calendar. *Gradually but inevitably,* your brain, body, heart and soul will thank you. We that are part of your human experience will thank you too! So What? So . . .

"RISE AND SHINE!"

You bought this book—free heart for you!

Practiced the Yamas and the Niyamas—specifically, Ahimsa (Be nice to yourself!)

Practiced Physical Yoga Asana

Practiced Bearing Witness

Had a professional massage

Had a home massage

Switched out paraben-laden lotion for oil or organic lotion

Listened to chill-out tunes in the car/subway

Used essential oils

Physically threw out or boxed up things that don't belong to you that are cluttering the space

Physically threw out low-self-worth clothing

Performed sage smudging

Physically organized living space to promote positivity

Brought fresh flowers into your home

Created elemental balance (maybe even a small altar, or personal sacred space)

Added a crystal to my space

Made use of mandala, yantra and sacred geometry

When tempted to eat a sweet, ate an organic, healthy version

Tried dehydrated greens powder

Tried a green juice or fresh fruit smoothie (no processed sugar!)

Checked out healthy prepared food services available in your neighborhood

Tried a healthy version of one of your favorite recipes

Looked into Ayurveda; Chinese Medicine; talked to a homeopath

Used supplements for my dosha (constitution)

Let go of mental space

Let go of cyber space

Made an "I am willing to let go . . ." list

Abstained from alcohol (despite the desire)

Abstained from caffeine (despite the desire)

Abstained from small-minded behaviors (despite the desire)

Engaged in social activity with loved ones (human)

Engaged in social activity with loved ones (animal)

Engaged in social activity with children or elders (human, heehee)

Spent time with the girls, just being girls

Practiced some form of Seva (Selfless Service)

Gave gratitude instead of attitude in public

Created a gratitude list

Sent a card, email or made a phone call thanking someone for something

Minded your mental patterns and caught an off-track thought

Used an affirmation

Signed up for a fun, online, happy thought resource

Practiced love, kindness, meditation

Sent a prayer, talked aloud or wrote a letter to someone who has passed

Abstained from totally psychotic break-up behavior (despite desire)

Practiced forgiveness mentally

Called, emailed, texted or snail-mailed a forgiveness greeting

Believed that **gradually but inevitably** you would rise and shine!

"Gradually but inevitably whatever you give love to is
going to thrive. Whatever you give love to is going
to just grow and blossom and be successful."

—MC Yogi

Namasté, Yogi!
Congratulations! Gold Star! A+!

Your reward (and motivator) is this Paul Teodo "centerfold." We picked Paul up at the YogaWorks on Main Street in Santa Monica. He was drooling over Sara Ivanhoe. We were drooling over him. I've seen many a small screen starlet slip out of side angle pose after getting a glance of Paul's *six-pack*. In addition to being a Chicago-raised, college-educated, licensed real estate broker, dedicated actor and delicious guitar player with manners, class, and cooking skills for miles, Paul is really hot. He's allowed us to objectify him (for the heartbroken girls, of course).

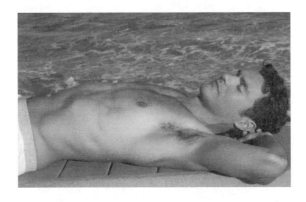

"Yoga is the most comprehensive form of wellness I have ever found. I am constantly amazed at how it has improved my life physically, mentally, and spiritually. I believe everyone should give it a try, and see the difference a regular practice can make in your life. And meditate!"

—PAUL TEODO, HEART THROB

CHAPTER 14

Love

"I look at the heart."

—Sridhar Silberfein, the Center for Spiritual Studies

"Time out!" the circulating nurse yelled loudly. All the staff in the surgical suite paused and directed their attention to the woman as she "identified the patient" asleep on the slab. The team listened intently, asked questions accordingly and went about their business preparing for the emergency quadruple by-pass.

Again, "Time out" the circulating nurse yelled loudly. All the staff in the surgical suite paused and directed their attention to the thoracic surgeon leaping into the room like a lightning bolt, good ol' Dr. Peterson donning his scrubs and red satin cape. Dr. Peterson takes over the second time out, recapping the medical background and then identifying the patient as an actual, living, feeling, human being "Claire Dewhurst. Sixty-two years old. Protestant. Husband is pacing around the waiting room. Only daughter is on a plane from California. Let's give her some good news when she lands." The entire team then takes a moment to "focus"—what we non-medical lay people might refer to as a "moment of silence" or even "setting the sankalpa." It would be a HIPAA violation for me to disclose much more about that moment; however, according to an off-duty, off-campus charge nurse under the promise of anonymity:

"It's a standard of care. It's a requirement that is adhered to for good reason. We obviously want to do the right thing, for the right patient, at the right time. For myself and for everyone I'm aware of on our team, even though we are diverse in our religious practices or our choice that our God is not necessarily confined to a church, our people start their day with prayer or their intention of just doing their best job for the other person. I think that's what secures people in doing what they do, because they know they are making their best effort. And a heart team knows that no matter how good any one individual is, it's not any one individual on the team, it's the team. And for our team, each individual has the choice to include their spiritual background and their faith in God as they see it and practice it. Sounds a little hokey in this day and age, but that's the reality."

Last December some friends and I threw Mariel Hemingway her surprise 50th birthday party. The next day I attended my Bhakti Yoga Shala Teacher Training Exam and thankfully, graduation. Like any good big sister-type, Sara Ivanhoe snapped photos, snuck in a secret flute of champagne, embarrassed me in front of my new friends, then dutifully drove me to the airport for my flight east. I'm still not great at planning ahead or remembering to use my airline miles. Swaha.

As I hopped out of her Prius, Sara (draped in Prada) gave me the requisite post-stress, pre-travel pep talk:

"You did great. You'll be great. You look great. You are great. And Ame?"

"Yeah?"

"Don't forget to do your practice."

"Thanks Ma," I answer, with an aggravated yet appreciative "I know" eye roll.

The six in-flight hours were spent in sadhana (spiritual practice). I had my hands in anjali mudra and set a sankalpa for a safe flight. I enjoyed healthy products for my senses. Made lists and said aloud some things I can let go of. Gave gratitude for all the amazing people who have made up this part of the adventure, forgave myself and others for the mistakes and mea culpas along the way. I did my mantra. I remembered that I may not feel like a perfect incarnation of the infinite today, however, gradually but inevitably the message I need to hear is always revealed. I recalled being at the bottom and feeling like love had forsaken me, like God forgot my phone number, wondering if my candle would ever be lit again, or if anyone even noticed I was sitting in the dark. Then I laughed, thinking about all the times I have felt that way before. Just when I think I won't survive, a wave of Grace rolls in from the infinite ocean, scoops me up and carries me safely to a strange shore—one that was ten times cooler than I had collaged into a vision board, or Google-bookmarked for a romantic rendezvous.

My plane safely lands in Jersey. Sue, Jim Jim Murphy and their girls cruise in to pick up Crazy Auntie Amy from California. Cue adorable Car Christmas Scene: stories of Santa, Rudolph, who's been naughty, who's been nice and the like. We arrive at the First Congregational Church of River Edge, the place where I first found out about this God guy three decades ago. Pilgrim Hall is abuzz with "Good News of a Great Joy" as the little angels, candle angels, shepherd angel and annunciation angel get on their glitter and gold. The pack of awkward teenage boys masquerading as kings and shepherds in silk robes and scratchy beards stumble around outside with their staffs, sheep and a few spliffs. Some things never change. Now too old and too tall to casually slip on an angel costume (although let's be honest—sometimes I still try), I enter the sanctuary, walk up the stairs and into the Manger. From here I have the great honor of narrating The Christmas Story. My favorite part is the verse "And Mary kept all of these things, pondering them in her heart."

It speaks of the time between the appearance of the annunciation angel, telling Mary that she is pregnant with the Son of God, and when she starts to show. That little baby bump later becomes known as Jesus Christ; perhaps the most well-known representation of love, gratitude, forgiveness and grace.

What would you do if an angel showed up and told you God was already inside you? Would you read yourself the riot act? Take another Ambien? Or ponder these things in your heart?

In Bhakti Yoga Shala, there is an altar to the patron deity of the heart, Hanuman. In the ancient Hindu epic *The Ramayana,* Hanuman embodies love, compassion and selfless service. Toward the conclusion of this 24,000-verse poem, the good guys win. The princess is rescued, the rightful prince regains his throne and Hanuman is awarded jewels for helping to restore peace in the land. The kingdom then doubts the dignity of his devotion. Hanuman is all action, all the time. He responds without the weight of words. He simply rips his chest open to reveal his truth—his beloveds, Sita and Ram, at home in his heart. **Hanuman knew love was already inside of him. We humans forget.**

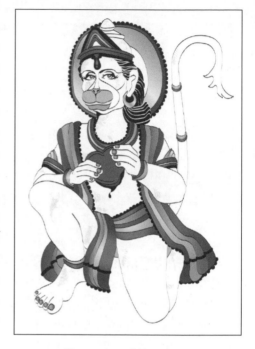

Illustration of Hanuman.

We cast stones, build walls and wage wars (even against ourselves).

I can tell you for a fact that when the second plane hit the world trade center and all the concrete, debris, paper, and people were showering down from the sky, no one was doubting each other's dignity, comparing religions, beliefs, sexual preference or political persuasions. They simply ran, screamed and then embraced their fellow man. No such comparisons were made when Stan was on casualty patrol in Fallujah; when my friend Michael Klein went to the Wailing Wall in Jerusalem; in the Preemie Unit of Cedars Sinai; or on the streets of Point Pleasant Beach, when Hurricane Sandy decimated the Jersey Shore.

In these moments of chaos, confusion, helplessness, hope and grief people grabbed one another's hands and got real. In the face of tragedy, private or public, all the bullshit stories we layer on top of ourselves fall away. What we're left with is our truth.

At Chris's funeral, the priest instructed us to lay a rose atop his casket and proceed to our cars. No one moved a muscle. There were about 400 people at that service, but I stood solo in the cemetery, sobbing—a scene all too standard to this particular group, in this particular cemetery.

I tried to lead the charge. Calm. Assertive. Hard. Fast. Defined, attainable goal. My *Jimmy Choos* got stuck in the graveyard grass. If my twenties taught me one thing, it's not to wear heels to a wake, funeral, or all-you-can-drink New Year's Eve Party. But when the pall bearing boys nervously beeped the car horn ten minutes too soon that morning, I heard the echo of an old scene from that one September: *"It's what he would have wanted me to wear,"* she said, *uncharacteristically strong.*

When our friend Coco made the *New York Times* Style Section and scored us the sample Choos, Chris was the one who sent the email around proudly announcing the news. He had the capacity and consciousness to genuinely be happy for other people, be present when you were talking, and remember details about your life and work that he had no tangible experience of, or way to relate to. Like knowing Fashion Week is in September just after his anniversary, just before his birthday. He made a note of it because it was important to Coco, which made it important to EZ-E, which made it important to Chris. A quality I thought rare "these days." I flashed through these thoughts while trying to wriggle the stem of the shoe out of the ground. The stem of the rose had now pricked my finger. *I'm stuck and I'm bleeding and I'm alone and this is just so unjust, what was the point of taking a person like this off the planet? How could God do this? To his new wife, to his best friend, to his grandmother, to his aunts, uncles, sisters, and the few hundred teammates, co-workers, neighbors and friends who have gathered here? This can't be happening. This isn't real. I can't breathe. I can't move and there is blood streaming out of my finger.* The drycleaner at The Malibu Country Mart already had me on her shitlist. She had sternly warned about coffee and Sharpie stains on silk, telling me if I bought a white coat again this winter she wasn't responsible for it. *She's going to be so pissed if I get blood all over this satin sheath, and then she won't do my alterations overnight anymore when I've booked a last-minute acting job, or steam my gown when I receive a day-of premiere invite. The tissues are soaked with snot and won't stop the blood that is now gushing and staining the Stella McCartney that cost a car payment. Fuck. This is not happening. We cannot be standing in this fucking cemetery together again. To bury another friend too young, too gifted, too special, too loved. I can't breathe. Everything is fuzzy. Is this what fainting feels like? Omg, I think I might be fainting. I'm not wearing any underwear, I can't faint here. Or anywhere for that matter, but I really cannot faint here and now. Do not faint! I knew better than to wear these shoes. Do not faint! You teach yoga, you know how to breathe, do it! Do not faint! Breathe! Breathe! Breathe!*

At that moment I felt a familiar arm around my waist. It was an old friend I hadn't spoken to since the band broke up. That summer down the shore about ten years ago when She . . . So I . . . So then she . . . so then I . . . Standing in a cemetery, it doesn't matter who said what to who, when. Who slept with who. Who didn't tell who that who slept with who, and all the other complications we come up with to build walls around ourselves.

No words were spoken, but the healing happened. In that moment we weren't rights and wrongs, he saids, she saids. We were just two souls, swimming in the fishbowl. The 21 grams of atman within the hridayam, the light that shines brightly, leading our way out of the darkness. From untruth to truth. From death to immortality. From "we had a falling-out" to the silently exchanged, "Apology accepted, now help me stop this bleeding, and get unstuck from the dirt (the mithya and the maya)."

When we're down on the ground trying to figure out what it all means, and our hearts are bruised and bloody, they crack wide open. It's a good time to get out all the gunk. Decide what is truly important. Who is best suited for your team. If you don't tidy up in there, how will you have room for your beloveds?

After Chris traveled to the great gig in the sky, and TS plowed through with the heartbreak hit and run, I took the whole season to spring-clean.

The lessons learned in losing someone from your starting line-up require time, space, and self-care. TS illuminated the pretty parts of myself that needed someone to spark them. Then he lit a Molotov cocktail and winged it at me from behind the safety of his computer screen.

In a thick Irish brogue, Jim Jim Murphy's ma, Maureen, mother of five, grandmother of ten, shakes a finger. "Practice what you preach." I can preach the aforementioned practices because when I received that awful email I didn't "Go Jersey" and get defensive, neck swinging around like Snooky after six sandwiches, ordering Sue's brothers-in-law to break TS's knee caps. I just felt so sad for him. I had told TS he was loving, lovable and loved by me. He responded in caps, "GET YOUR SHIT TOGETHER, DUDE." How much spring cleaning do you think his heart needs? Ooppph.

Let's all send him some love, and maybe the toll-free number for Merry Maids. Hint: It's 1-855-HAN-UMAN. When you call it up, you can hear the most cherished chant celebrating the space within the Heart, the Hanuman Chalisa—a beautiful 40-verse prayer that is chanted continuously in the hills of Kainchi, India. It played on repeat while Govindas built Bhakti Yoga Shala, while Ram Dass wrote "Be Here Now," while Krishna Das taught us all "Gradually but inevitably," while special souls gathered in satsang on Bhakti Fest mornings, while I told my tales of Heartbreak, and in innumerable temples, ashrams, hills, valleys, homes and hearts internationally.

The Hanuman Chalisa concludes with the following verse:

"Keejai natha hridaya mahan dera"—

"Lord, make your home in my heart."

During the down-on-the -ground, spring-clean season, I dusted the part of the temple that he could make his home in. I got the gunk out by tearing down the walls, letting go of large cardboard boxes too old and too heavy to hold. I swept out the broken glass caused by Biggie's lack of bravery and TS's time bomb. I chose my team and thought of an old phrase the sailors still use: "Have faith, tides change." I practiced my sadhana and paddled out stronger than the set before. Hopefully grace goes easy on me in the next swell. I've invited God into my heart.

My gothed-out, atheist, punk rock drummer friend has been bugging me about a sound bite—what God means to me in two sentences or less. I can't do it. I don't know. What I do know is how I felt when my mom came out of surgery alive; what Joshua Tree sounds like at night; Kim's face when Bruce Springsteen wished her a Happy Birthday from the Stadio Olimpico Stage; holding my nephew for the first time; the sight of Fourth of July Fireworks falling down over Venice Beach rooftops; watching Sue sparkle when Jim Jim Murphy "kissed the bride"; the exaltation of the "Amens" from within the Harlem churches; the silence of a sky-diving free-fall high above the Rocky Mountains; the clip-clop of high heels walking down Wall Street; the thrill of sitting atop a speeding concert-bound bus on a country road in the middle of nowhere; group-hugging my girlfriends at our high school graduation, knowing nothing would ever be the same; the belly laughs and bad bangs my cousins and I have shared over the years; the precision and beauty with which my grandmother set a dinner table; standing on my dad's feet as he danced; my mom's kisses; my MA's hugs; and the space that is created when I just sit quietly on my yoga mat and allow myself to be loved—to feel the love that was already there inside of me this whole time.

It's always the last place you look isn't?

Of course, I can never just contemplate something solo. When I get excited, I become like a three-year-old, high on chocolate and running around hoping everyone is as excited as I am. Bouncy Castle—AAAHHHHH!!

So, I asked my cast of characters what they thought about love. I give you my own personal version of the *Scrooged* finale. For the full experience, please download or play from YouTube:

• Jackie DeShannon's "Put A Little Love in Your Heart"

• Jai Uttal's "Maha Mantra/Help"

• MC Yogi's, "Give Love"

Play it loud.

Love is meant to be heard, seen, touched, tasted, and blown wide open by.

LOVE IS . . .

Sri Dharma Mittra
"Love is the pure ultimate joy that flows from the source of love: the Supreme Self."

Shiva Baum—Partner/Bender Music Group, Los Angeles, CA
"Love is an exquisite paradox. We invest almost all of our energy in chasing, pursuing, searching and chasing it yet again . . . only to finally come home to our own heart to find the love we were searching for was actually there all along. Much of our deepest internal suffering is learning to live with this . . . Learning that true love doesn't exist in loving someone else, but in learning to love ourselves."

Stephen Nemeth—Rhino Records
"Love is rare but mercifully not unattainable and when real, it's brilliant!"

Ronald A. Alexander, Ph.D.—Author, *Wise Mind, Open Mind*
Love is allowing the dissolution of the ego to enter the Heart's fire where the Divine essence purifies the separateness by dissolving I (me) mine, and through the ashes of one's divinity we merge into the sacred space of endless streaming Bhakti flow. It is in that space of infinite and everlasting oneness that we discover the selfless energy of true giving. Love is both letting go of our fears and learning to give without thought of return. The more we give love the more we are enshrined in love. In this space of purity we learn that love is love!

Donna Morong—Casting Director / *10 Things I Hate About You, The Princess Diaries, Gone Baby Gone*

Love connects us to each other; love does not judge but accepts with eyes wide open. It changes as we change and as we grow and experience our lives. It makes us forget ourselves as we become whole for a moment, warmed with a feeling devoid of all boundaries. It is a connection to a lover, a baby, a student, a patient, a friend, a relative. It can be sexual or it can be chaste. It drives us and it calms us. It is a force of goodness but it can also be used for evil. It is an idea and it is pure feeling. It's in the mind but it warms the body. It's what "makes the world go 'round."

Amanda Borja— Team Fit Training, Venice, CA

Love is always changing and growing, just like my belly! It is putting another's needs before my own. Love is being patient and waiting for joy that is to come. It is so deep that I think I cannot fathom it . . . at least not until the day arrives and our baby is born.

Nina Rao

"Love is the space that holds the whole world; where we can accept and give equally with no conditions; where we are all one; Love is the space we always want to be in. They say that it is our true nature, so we can actually find it— imagine that!"

Bryan Kest—Founder of Donation Based Yoga at PowerYoga, Santa Monica, CA

"You don't find love, it finds you."

Daniel Paul—Tabla Player

"Amy, now that's quite a request, but coming from you I should've expected it. Love to me , it's felt quite warmly in the heart when certain things line up, fears and neediness disappear, unconditional acceptance reigns supreme, and in the case of partnership love, you still just can't get enough of each other! There ya go! Life in the fast lane . . ."

Jaimie Hilfiger—Model/Designer
"Love is life's greatest luxury."

Peter Shapiro—The Wetlands/The Brooklyn Bowl /The Jammys
"Love is something you cannot describe with words."

David Cassidy—Producer, Cabin Creek Films
"Love is the beauty that comes with discovering things for the first time all over again with your child."

Mark Mancina—Composer, *The Lion King, Training Day, Speed*
"Love is . . . complete and total surrender. Perhaps the most impossible task for a human being. And yet, in that regard, the most challenging task of all."

Devin Rich—Associate Producer, NBC's *Parenthood,* Burbank, CA
"Love is exactly what you want it to be. :)"

Kelli McCarty—Photographer/Actress/Model, Los Angeles, CA
"LOVE is how my Rescue animals look at me after I've saved them from the shelter."

David Newman—Kirtan Artist, Philadelphia, PA
"Love is to forgive, accept, understand, and truly care. It is the expression of a connection between two souls that is based upon fearlessness and non-judgment and is the spontaneous outpouring of an open heart which sees no difference between itself and the 'other'."

Patrick McArney—Captain Tony's Saloon, Key West, Florida
"Captain Tony had thirteen children with eight different women, five wives, and when he passed away at ninety-two the kids were ages twenty-two to seventy-two. Now that's love. Ah ha ha ha ha"

Grandma Noy—Age 93
"Love can't be described by words, but proven by action. Love can't be written in song, and by action smitten. Let's work on the world, and give love a whirl."

Rae Ray—Venice Beach Skate Park Photographer
"Love is unconditional and has no opposite. The most precious thing you can give someone you love is not something you can buy; it's your true presence, your full attention."

Patricia Karpas—Gaiam TV
"Love is the energy you put into the world with every breath, in every moment."

Julie Schubert—Casting Director, *Footloose,* New York, NY
"Love is a donut from the corner bodega at 3 am on a work day because you woke up and had a craving and he didn't want you to go out so late in the crappy neighborhood you rent an apartment in."

Todd Stoops—Keyboardist, Raq & Kung Fu
"Love is hearing your wife's voice in your child's laughter, seeing her eyes sparkle inside your son's when he's giggling, and feeling your heart swell up inside of your chest to the point of bursting when you imagine this life without them . . ."

Jamie Buckner—Production Coordinator, *Men in Black III*
"Love is fearless, unconditional comfort."

Antoinette Lee—Designer, Antoinette Lee Designs
"Love is laughter, luck, and the endless feeling of butterflies in your stomach."

DJ GOLDBERG—McG's Wonderland Sound and Vision, Hollywood, CA
"Love is whatever you choose to make of it, but, to me, it's a feeling that I
associate with comfort, integrity, emotion, joy, humor, and most of all, respect.
You just know. eek"

Stefano Tortora—Mechanic, Emerson, NJ
"Love is drinking a bud can, watching the Yankees, with my dog Mattingly."

Terri Craft—Juice Magazine, Venice Beach, CA
"LOVE is everything. Love is all-consuming passion, loyalty, sacrifice and
devotion. It wakes you up in the morning and can keep you up all night long.
It's the feeling you have when everything else fades into the background and
love is all that matters."

Kim Surowicz—Feature Film and Documentary Producer
"Love is the feeling you get in your gut when the guy of your dreams walks in a
room.
Love is friends showing up when you don't expect them to.
Love is baking cookies and mailing them across the country.
Love is knowing that you're never alone.
Love is a handwritten letter.
Love is an amazing sunset.
Love is the giggling of a child whose been caught by the tickle monster.
Love is doing someone's laundry for them.
Love is yoga . . . especially after a rough few weeks!"

Caspar Poyck—Conscious Life Taster
"Life will always bring change. Love is the ability to value it all; the easy and the hard. Love is accepting truth and trusting it."

Jason Wachob—Mind-Body-Green
"Love is accepting others for who they are. Nothing more, nothing less."

Naganath—The Retreat at Two Rivers, Costa Rica
"Love is the Glowing Vibrating Manifestation of It All!"

Mark Dembinsky—Manager, Starbucks, Bradenton, FL
"Love is never feeling obligated, but always being accountable."

Rob Augusta—Rocket Scientist, El Segundo, CA
"Love is astronomical alignment plus the collection of your shared moments."

Dennis Gubbins—Comedian, Los Angeles, CA
"Love is like a box of chocolates—once you start eating them you just can't stop, but then you get sick. Is it Valentine's Day yet?"

Mary Firestone—Los Angeles, CA
"Love is giving up the idea of perfection. Of letting someone see you—all of you and love you for it, and accepting another person as they are. There is no "perfect man" or "perfect woman." I think people hold out for this idealized partner that doesn't exist. Love is not supposed to be blissful and passionate all the time. It is messy and challenging and that's the point, to grow and expand. That is love's ultimate gift."

Genevieve Walker—Violinist, San Francisco, CA
"Love is a thread of connection at times electric, at times silent, that threads through experience and time. This thread of connection is what gives you the strength and fuel to traverse the beautiful and difficult terrain of life. Through . . . Love, loss, beauty and decay."

Thomas Duggan—Venice Cruisers
"I JUST LOVE 2 LOVE!" ;)-

Ashley Cook—Ash and Dan's
"Love is having a nook."

Cosibella—Team Mom, Kauai, HI
"Love is the pull, the yearning, the passionate journey into Self, yet beyond Self. Love is a surrendering and unbounding of the compassionate heart, revealing the deepest, most sacred pulse that invites us to serve, celebrate, and honor the highest good of all. Love is an action that requires courage, humility, faith and discipline. Love is the strength in our vulnerability; the promise held in each breath. Love is the juiciness and lusciousness of life.
And I love you."

I asked a certain favorite Wall Streeter of mine, "What Is Love?" He responded with the following email:

Wow. From dark to deep. Under an agreement of anonymity, I will share as follows:

1. Omni present thought . . . first thought as you awake, last thought before you fall asleep
2. A sense of anticipation that is indescribable. The racing of the heart, the sweating of the palms.

3. The gut reaction at the mere mention of the person's name.

4. The gasp, or utter lack of focus on anything but him/her as they enter a room.

5. The scanning of a room as you enter, in hopes of finding him or her without further delay.

6. The sharing of your most intimate thoughts without concern or hesitation.

7. The emptiness when apart, and the lack of desire to remediate the emptiness.

8. The tone of your voice, and overall attitude change when you answer the phone, knowing it's them calling.

9. The acceptance of their shortcomings or missteps, and full reciprocation of such.

10. The first person you think of when you have good news to share. The person you want by your side when bad news occurs.

11. The disproportionate amount of time spent looking for a gift . . . not expensive, but meaningful.

12. The memories conjured up from a particular song, or perhaps a food or cocktail.

13. The incessant whispering of his or her name, even when you are not together.

14. The full understanding of your senses, from sight, smell, taste, hearing, touch . . . a heightened level of awareness you never dreamed possible.

Not sure any of these things "define" love, but they certainly are components of such. If you're lucky enough to experience it once in your life, you'll know it. Hopefully you're with the one who stirs these emotions. Life could be unbearable, if not.

A moment later I received another email from him:

Should add . . . love of a child has totally different implications, but can be equally powerful. But love of a dog is the purest form of love. LOL . . . Totally reciprocated and unconditional.

Travis Eliot—Power Yoga, Santa Monica, CA
"What is LOVE? It's not fear or anger; it's not comparing or judging. LOVE is what makes a child smile. LOVE is a stranger helping another without expecting anything in return. LOVE is what creates, sustains and even dissolves life. It's infinite, boundless, eternal and what fuels ALL of creation."

Ara Khorozian—Lawyer/Son/Dad/Brother
"Love is understanding we are on this planet to serve and live for our families."

Nicole De La Rosa—Gaiam TV
"Love is the illuminated spark between your soul and the world."

Abigail Lewis—*Whole Life Times*
"Love is recognizing a need in someone else and responding to that need with a pure heart. Warm, fuzzy feelings are just a bonus."

I called Mo the Yoga Dog's mom, Amanda G:
    Amanda G: Mo, Amy is on the phone for you. What is love?
    Mo: "Aaare roooaaar rooooarrroouuuhhhh"

Coco
"When you open the door and you hear 'click click click click' and it's your dog running to you because he/she is so happy to see you, it's the only true unconditional love that exists."

I had dharma talk with my good friend Bodhi Gorman, age 2.
Amy: Hey Bode, What's the heart?
Bodhi: "LOVE!"
Amy: What Is Love?
Bodhi: "I love you!"
Amy: (Heart melts) Awww, I love you too, Bud.

Then he threw his arms around my neck and we danced to the beat of his
dad's bass, and his mom's beautiful voice from backstage.

Mary Arden Collins—Singer
"Love is warm. Love is safe. Love is free . . .
Free flowing connection from one heart to another.
Love is the net that is there to catch you when you fall.
Love inspires you to be your best . . . and want the best for another.
Love is sparkly."

Jai ma—Wah!
"Love is coherent energy, invisible to the naked eye and present in the
molecules of all living things. Love can only be felt through expression. You
have to be it, say it, show it, do something as an act of love in order to feel it."

Daniel Levy—Sotheby's International Real Estate
"Love is when all of the issues your partner has are worth it, because no one is
perfect and everyone has something. I remember having girlfriends with the
most trivial of issues and in some selfish way I did not want to deal with them
or care that much. I knew I was in love with the person I was with because
none of her issues, no matter how big or small, would faze me."

Gloria Dibiase—Jerry Garcia Art Archive
"LOVE! A beautiful concept & a beautiful word! I read many years ago in a

book about 'Thoughtforms' that the word LOVE, when spoken or thought makes one of the most beautiful forms above the head of the speaker/ thinker! So to make this world a more beautiful, peaceful, happy world, we should think & say that word more often! What the World Needs Now, Is LOVE, SWEET LOVE!"

Michael Byrne (Didj)—Casa Barranca, Ojai, CA
"Love is a vibration that we feel with our heart. When it comes to emotion, humans can be likened to prisms. We literally leave rainbows of emotions in our wake. Pure love exists unfiltered. During powerful moments or through, careful self-examination we begin to see through the walls of our illusory self. We catch scattered glimpses through the spider-webbed window of our ego. We hear distant thunder and know—even though our eyes are closed—that somewhere there is lightning. Love is a vibration we feel with our heart and it glues the whole perfectly fractured mandalic world together."

Mom
"In my experience, love is the quickening of your heartbeat when the man you love is near. It is the feeling you have when looking into the eyes of your baby for the very first time and knowing that you will do anything for that child. Love is a mother who makes you feel like you can accomplish anything and shows by example how to live with grace and dignity. It is grieving the loss of a parent and knowing that one day you will be reunited. Love is the laughter you share with family and friends. It is the bond that binds family together through the thick and thin of life. It is the pride you feel when the successes of life bless you and the failures of life try to bring you down. It is supporting the dreams of a family member or friend and expecting nothing in return. Love, undying love, is what I feel for my husband and daughter and for the joy they have given me and continue to give me. It is the pride I feel for Jessica, Jorie, Nicole, Zach, Liam, Kaia and Quinn and the joy they bring to my life. Love is the special bond I share with my sister and brother-in-law and the memories we have. It is that special feeling I have for Kerrith, Arax and Lisa, not sisters by birth but sisters nonetheless. Love is the wonderful feeling that fills my life daily and I thank God for being so very blessed."

Laura Amazzone—Priestess, Venice, CA
"Surrendering to the Great Mystery of Divinity within oneself and in another. Opening to the ever-flowing energies of expansion and contraction, joy and sorrow, separation and union. Trusting the unknown. That is Love."

Jai Uttal—Grammy-nominated Kirtan Artist
"When my son was born, really for the first time, I experienced the feeling of putting someone else higher then myself. I always felt that way toward God, and my Guru (Maharaj-ji–Sri Neem Karoli Baba), but it's different with humans. Suddenly I felt like my whole being was—take care of this other being and not out of responsibility or obligation, but out of complete, complete love and desire to do so, not desire to get something back. That has just continued and it has completely changed my relationship to Bhakti, to devotion, where it used to be about an experience; you know, that I would be experiencing, something like an ecstasy or a longing. Then it wasn't about my experience, it was about his. I would sing it for his experience, for his enjoyment, fulfillment, his ecstasy. That translates back to God, and Guru. In my case, rather than going from love of God, and that trickling down to human, it worked actually the opposite way, that the human love increased my spiritual; it's all spiritual, but it increased my love for God, for my Guru."

Chris Morro
"The Beatles were right on target when they sang, 'All You Need Is Love.' The purest form of love requires no 'other.' It is a gift of Grace, where the soul is able to feel it's innate connectedness to all things. In this state of love there is no requirement for another to make us happy. We are even able to love those who hate us, because when blessed with this Grace, it allows us to see the ultimate reality behind God's play. As my guru often said, 'All One.'"

Dan Steinberg—Photographer, Portland, Oregon
"To answer your question . . . Love, in the spiritual sense, is what we feel or become aware of when we quiet down enough to connect to our true divine nature. Ram Dass says it perfectly with his mantra 'I am loving awareness.' Love is our true nature, it emanates from within us effortlessly. Our job is to quiet our ego mind enough to experience it fully."

Vernoy (Nunu) Paolini—My Godmother
"Nothing exists between the depths of the ocean and the infinite reaches of the universe that can compare with the love for my grandbabies. That kind of love is all encompassing, ever-present, and lives in the sparkle of an eye. My beautiful grandbabies are 'double-decker' love—child of my child—a reflection of those who have passed—a perfect memory of the tiny little hands I held of my own children and that fleeting innocence so quickly gone . . . a gift from above that I really don't feel worthy of because who could possibly be so precious and so significant to deserve such joyous happiness?

". . . and then she says spontaneously, smiling sweetly, encircling my face with her little hands, 'Oh . . . my perfect NuNu!'. . . and there is no denying that I know love."

Mike Ponce—Sneaker Designer, El Segundo, CA
Love is empathy
Love is a big old smile
Love is Gratitude
Love is being kind to others
Love comes and goes
Love more live more

John Dewhurst—My dad
"Love is when your daughter calls you 'Dad' for the first time, on Father's Day."

Mrs. Heinzinger—Director of Christian Education, First Congregational
Church of River Edge/ producer of the Christmas Pageant
"Love is conceived in friendship, fueled by passion, nurtured and sustained
by mutual respect, honesty and laughter."

Dan Wilf—Yoganonymous
"I used to be in love. I still am—but I used to be also."

Sean Gesell—VP of Production, Zucker Entertainment
"Love is wanting to spend time with your significant other, even when they're
being poopy . . ."

Kiko Marra—Soundboard Dude, John Fogerty/Jurassic 5
"Love is unconditional. It's like when you're 16 and you're yelling at your
parents, but they still love you anyway."

Cindy Kokesch, PA
"Love is energy we feel when we connect to another by being open and
allowing them to see/share/experience into our soul and, vice versa, we are
graced with their trust to see/share/experience their true deep soul energy."

Kaia Gallagher—Age 4, New Jersey
"Love means kisses and hugs."

Liam Gallagher—Age 7
"Love means hugs and kisses and the heart."

Jennifer Quail—Bicoastal Writer
She knows she knows me. It's that recognition that makes it so hard; that same beaming smile that has met me my entire life.

She knows she knows me; knows I've been around a while, that she watched me grow up, braided my hair, told me bedtime stories.

She knows she knows me but isn't sure why or what my name might be. But she knows to smile, to take my hand as she drifts back to sleep and say she loves me.

She knows she knows me because something in her heart still recognizes love that's true.

Richard Wegman—Chief Operating Officer, Global Green USA
"Love is the source of the universe, the source of all things. In the beginning there was God and She yearned, that yearning is Love, Our love for God is to answer that call, our love for each other and our love for the planet is the same. Love is our reason for being, it is what we are here to do. Loka Samasta Sukhino Bhavantu!"

Courtenay Brandt—Creative Director/Stylist, Los Angeles, CA
"Love is . . . fearlessly letting yourself go to the unknown and finding everything you dreamed of and things you didn't even know you wanted."

Steve Glick—The Glick Agency, Santa Monica CA
"Pure love is how you feel about your child."

Narayan Mandir Zalben
"l o v e, it seems as our limited perception allows, that it can be only felt. dreams are to be lived, even while witnessing reality as truth, the endless journeys of all souls are perceived through this portal we call love . . . it can be manifest, as, countless forms and deity, while being unmanifest as the shadow that is cast by the presence of our soul . . ."

Denise Kaufman—Bassist, squatting advocate, Ma
"You don't find love—you offer love."

Kia Miller—Kundalini Yoga Expert
"Love is:
At the deepest level we are ananda, bliss, we are love, we are connected through the subtlest vibration that does not recognize separation. In this place there is no fear, no resistance, just pure surrender, acceptance, deep compassion and a feeling of being connected to everyone and everything. From this place all is possible. Love is light, it is healing, it is compassion, it is the infinite space within and without. When we are living in love we see life from the perspective of abundance and living grace. Love connects us."

Tom Dagnino—Screenwriter/Alcon Entertainment
"Love is...a form of circular logic."

Kirsten Sheridan—Writer/In America
"Love is letting go. Letting go of self, of ego, of want, of demands. Love is letting go and setting free." X

Jason Gorman—Copywriter (and dad), New York, NY
"Love is sitting through anything on ice and pretending to enjoy yourself."

Tom Tobin—AD/ *The Good Wife,* NYC
"The bliss of a moment, the joy of a day. The passion that fuels the happiness. The excitement to take the next step. The love."

Sarah Thompson—Designer/CEO, Five Feather Clothing and Accessories, London
I don't think that love itself can be described—it lives beyond words outside of linear time and asks to be felt, experienced and lived.

Love does not understand limitation—so when we try to distil it into words it feels a little like trying to chase sunlight into a glass jar—the more that we try to contain its essence, the more it dances away from us.

It is only when we shift our gaze slightly that we catch a clear glimpse of love's beauty in the spectrum of its reflections—the many faces that it inhabits and illuminates in our lives and the emotions, hopes, actions and dreams that it inspires.

Tara M. Sheahan—Mom/Founder, Conscious Global Leadership/Lover of this world, Carbondale, CO
"Love is the wisdom to be in it, or out of it.'

Dave Stringer—Kirtan Wallah
    "Love is the bearing
    I hold in my heart
    a compass unerring,
    the goal and the start
    the light of a beacon
    when all hope is lost
    the sight I am seeking,
    the ocean to cross"

I asked my best friend Sue. The phone conversation went like this:
Amy: Suze, what is love? ??
Sue: Love is . . . hold on a sec. What, Em? Okay, mommy is on the phone, just

a minute. Ame? What were you saying? How's it going with the book? Wait, hold on a sec.

Ava, take the bottle, baby, that's a good girl. So, was the date as fun as you had hoped? I'm sorry, I mean the book. How's it going? Ohmigod, that's great. I'm so happy for you.

Wait hold on a sec, Jim just got home. Hi hon, dinner is on the table, I'm just feeding the baby, Emma is washed up, the thank you note for my parents is on the table and Mike and Nicole's wedding gift too. Please sign your name to the cards. Thanks.

Ame? So, are you coming home for the wedding? Oh great, the kids will be so happy to see you. What are you going to wear? You always look great in that. I'm not sure what I'm going to wear because . . . Emma, do not hit your sister. Do you hear me? Mimi is inside. We'll see her in a little while. Yes, Pop Pop too. [The newborn starts screaming] There, there, it's okay baby, it's okay, Mommy's here.

Amy: Suze, I'll let you go. Love you.

Sue: Love you too. Emma, I said do not hit your sister! Do you hear me? Jim, can you do something please? That's all right, Ava, Mommy's here. Mommy's here.

Jim Jim Murphy—Sue's husband, Emma and Ava's dad, NJ

Love is packing/unpacking and moving four different times during a hurricane and power outage to make sure your wife and two daughters are safe. Love is having a bad day and then have it melt away when your daughter yells, 'DADDY!!!!" as loud as she can and jumps into your arms.

Love is watching your wife go through a new illness while pregnant and praying all day and night that she's going to be all right. Love is looking at your newborn child and not being able to lose a smile for days. Love is remembering past loved ones and seeing them in your children. Love is looking at your wife and wondering where she gets the time to do anything. Love is picking up your loved one's best friend in Harlem because you'll do anything to see that particular smile.

Keli Lalita Dasi—Mantrology
We are all eternally tiny sparks of the Divine, who is the supreme Source of love. So it is our birthright to possess perfect love. But much of the time, temporary material nature steals our loving potency from us. When it is reawakened, and there are so many ways for that to happen, we are able to again be completely humble, to give of ourselves with no expectations. We are able to overcome tremendous difficulty with ease. To be forgiving. To honor ourselves with radical acceptance and compassion, and to allow that same compassion and acceptance to radiate from our hearts to our loved ones. And even to those beings and people and situations that challenge us.

Giving birth at home to my three children holds the great teaching of the meaning of love. Never have I experienced such pain and intensity on a physical, and to some degree mental level, and never have I been so ready, willing and JOYFUL to do it! It was so unbelievably challenging and yet so wildly wonderful and so worth it. And I know that I would take a bullet for my husband or children without so much as batting an eyelash. That to me is love. Utter, joyful, surrender. Total humility, and no expectations.

Dr. David Rosenberg—Plastic Surgeon, Beverly Hills, CA
"Love is the strongest of bonds between two people; it is knowing you would do anything for the other, no matter the cost."

Izzy Shurte—Yoga teacher/Counseling Psychology Graduate Student, Asheville, NC
"Love loves you for all your shining strengths . . . and gently nudges you to examine your dark and weak places."

Chris Roy—Co-Founder and Tribal Leader at Namaste Interactive
"Love is what I saw the first time I looked into the eyes of my little boy. It was at that moment, that I realized Love is a grand and beautiful truth that lives at the core of our being. For me, it was the reflection in the unfiltered and pure gaze of a new born baby's eyes that awakened the knowing that we all share this boundless and eternal gift."

Jayon Anthony
"Love is an action verb—it's like magic!"

Cameron Albergo—Fort Lee, NJ
"The definition of love varies wildly from individual to individual. For some, it is an experience of feeling, for some it is an experience of thought, and for some it is never experienced at all."

Jason McHugh
"Love is like a big beautiful wave that you ride to glory with your new best friend for as long as possible . . .

Now that I am married, it's all about how to stay on that wave by making maneuvers for two while enjoying the sweet moves of my wife and, on occasion, happily coming to the rescue!"

Lisa Barrett—Executive, Peas and Carrots TV and Film
"Love is knowing that everything you are—morally, emotionally, and physically—whether it's your best day or your worst day will never scare him off, nor will he try to change you because to him you are 'perfect.' And he is 'perfect' to you."

Suzy Shelton—Manager of Maha Yoga, Brentwood, CA
"Love is the conscious choice to enjoy and feel gratitude for every moment, person, thing, situation."

Felicia Tomasko—Editor in Chief, *Find Bliss* and *LA Yoga*
"Love may be one of the hardest words to define in the English language. It's a

sense of surrender as well as a chance for confrontation and danger, adventure, sanctuary, and transformation. It is a conundrum and paradox—wild abandon and selfless giving. On whatever level we choose it, it is the great gift of this human life."

Zachary Carberry—Dad/Husband/Son/Communications Expert, Austin, Texas
"Love is an action, not a word and should be a core motivator behind every human interaction. Love is recognizing that one is truly vulnerable, wide open. One embraces this vulnerability, nurtures it. This is a shared experience, realized when one gazes upon another. One fosters this shared vulnerability and realizes that this LOVE, this undeniable connection will last forever, throughout suffering, happiness, joy and despair. LOVE will always be present. If the sadness overwhelms you, LOVE will fuel your soul through the pain. If you shed tears of joy, LOVE will be there to accentuate the jubilation. Love is recognizing the faults in others and accepting those faults. Love is how our souls communicate with one another."

Michelle Li—Journalist, Coastal Carolinas
"Love is unconditional. When you love someone, you really want the best for them, even if it's not you. When they love you back, you'll love them even when you want to poke their eyes out with a fork."

Bill Steinkamp—Editor, *Out of Africa*
"Love is seeing the world again thru my two and a half-year-old grandson's eyes, delicious!!!"

Scott Hecker—Supervising Sound Editor/ Designer, Universal Studios, Burbank, CA
"Inevitably we all experience both heartbreak and love in our lives. My heart was first broken when I was 21 after getting a 'Dear Scott' letter from my first love who I'd been with three and a half years . . . all good things come in time .

. . 27 years later we were reunited at our 30th high school reunion and have been sharing our lives together ever since . . .the script couldn't have been written any better!"

Joe McHugh—Artist
"The unknown awaits your kisses."

Shari Johnson—Author/ Editor/Grandmother, Odessa, TX
"Love is letting go of your expectations from others. A hard-learned lesson!"

The Other Deepak—Producer/Composer/Musician/Teacher/Universal Polymath, Malibu, CA
"Love . . .
All of existence is this essence, from the most complex to the most simple forms of matter and spirit. The indescribable space between the space, connecting it all together with infinite energy and infinite intelligence. Quantum God particles that contain the gamut of space, time, emotion, thought, past, present, and future. All of the realms of science, spirituality, art, history, mathematics, creations of nature and creations of man. The humble work of a farmer and the calculations of a rocket scientist, the smile of a wise old soul, and the laugh of every enlightened young child. The relationship of a human with another human, a friendship, lover, a child and a parent, and a human's relationship with that all purveying force that encompasses it all. The feeling, the concept, the idea, and that which cannot be explained, as it is beyond our 3-dimensional existence . . . 'Tis Love."

Gretchen Wallace—Founder & President, Global Grassroots, Hanover, NH
"I would actually like to share the definition that I learned from my spiritual teacher, Jessica Dibb, as it deeply resonates with me:
    'Unconditional Love is the unrelenting desire to respond to the highest need for awakening in the self and the other.'"

A parade of singers, drums and symbols marched along the ave at Sunset.

Amy: Vish!

(He couldn't hear me over all the hoopla.)

Amy: Vish! Bali! Dhanya! Vrinda! Kish! Vira!

(They couldn't hear me over all the hoopla.)

Amy: Hey! You guys! Wait up! I have an important question for you!!!

(They stopped and stared. It went silent.)

Amy: What Is Love?

(They did not pause, exchange an eye glance or any other signal that would indicate "Aaaand-aaaaa-one-two-three-four" they just BURST into song, singin'):

> *Hare Krishna*
> *Hare Krishna*
> *Krishna Krishna*
> *Hare Hare*
> *Hare Rama*
> *Hare Rama*
> *Rama Rama*
> *Hare Hare*
> *!!!!!!!!!!!!!!!!!!!!*

Radha Baum
September 23, 1971:
It felt like I had waited all my life to meet Maharajji, and here I was, actually with Him, receiving all the Love I always wished for, longed for, yet it was more than that. Unconditional Love was beyond what I ever experienced or imagined. K.K. Sah, one of the Indian Devotees, used to say that 'Maharajji stretches your capacity for Love.' I couldn't wait to be around Him during the days, and at night I dreamed of Him.

However one day, feeling exhausted and miserable, I stayed behind at the hotel, while it seemed all the other westerners had gone to the temple where Maharajji was. I didn't want to go and was determined not to, though this made no sense to me. There was a knock at the door, Krishna Das came in and asked what I was running from. Confused, I didn't know what to reply. 'It's the Love,' he said. 'The Love is so much we cannot bear it. All impurities come out in us.'

Soon afterward we left for the temple, and once again I was covered by the blanket of Maharajji's Love.

Rob Sidon—Editor, *Common Ground Magazine,* San Francisco, CA
Two quotes from Amma (Sri Mata Amritanandamayi):

"In this universe it is love that binds everything together. Love is the very foundation, beauty and fulfillment of life."

"Children, love can accomplish anything and everything. Love can cure diseases. Love can heal wounded hearts and transform human minds. Through love one can overcome all obstacles. Love can help us renounce all physical, mental and intellectual tensions and thereby bring peace and happiness."

BTW, I asked Biggie and TS to contribute their thoughts on what "Love is . . ."
    Biggie declined to comment.
    TS said he would "ruminate" and get back to me. He didn't—shocking!

AGGIE
I asked Schmag, "What is love?" She looked at me, resigned: "I have to solve your problems now too? All right . . ." (She jumped on the couch, crawled into the tiny space in my lotus-posture-lap and snuggled in. Now that's love.)

Mukti Silberfein—Bhakti Fest Producer
"Love is being in the Bhav at Bhakti Fest!"

"And love says, 'I will take care of you'
to everything that is near."
—Hafiz

A prayer for all those we love,
who traveled on during this leg of the journey:
Shyamdas, Maureen Murphy, MCA, Larry Schultz, Gypsy, Keith Page, Geoffrey Gordon, Aaron Garfinkle, Kevyn Aiken

❦   *In Loving Memory*   ❦

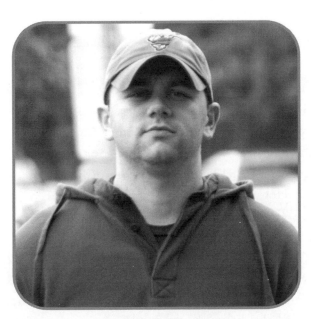

CHRIS MILLER
September 23, 1980 to March 25, 2012

About the Author

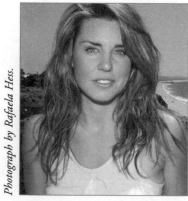

Photograph by Rafaela Hess.

Amy V. Dewhurst began her career as an extra on *Law and Order: Special Victims Unit* (half-clothed in Central Park during a New York City Winter). After recovering from pneumonia and the non-sag wages, she learned filmmaking while working on the production staffs of legends Sydney Pollack and Martin Scorsese. Dewhurst decided if she could wrangle 1,200 hungry extras through hair, make-up, wardrobe and United Nations Security (in a mini-skirt, reporting to set directly from her cocktail waitressing shift), she could probably do anything. Amy assisted director Kirsten Sheridan (*In America*) on Warner Brother's *August Rush* and later joined the development and production team of producer Richard B. Lewis (*Backdraft*).

The fast-paced film industry lifestyle led Amy to a disciplined yoga practice—she has since helmed Sara Ivanhoe's yoga and lifestyle company, Yoganation; Mariel Hemingway's health, wellness and production company, M. Hemingway Heritage; and has produced conscious content for Oasis Television.

Amy is a contributing writer for *Origin* magazine, *LA Yoga & Ayurveda* magazine, *Common Ground* magazine and *The Free Venice Beachhead* newspaper. She is currently writing her first feature film, is in development on a television pilot showcasing practical philanthropy globally, and produces Bhakti Fest, "the spiritual Woodstock of the decade." She ascribes to the philosophy of her teacher, Sri Mata Amritanandamayi: "Just Love and Serve."